# RICH DOCS

*Triple Your Practice Revenue*

By
Nicholas Shawn Chavez

Mr. Nicholas Shawn Chavez

No part of this publication may be reproduced, distributed or transmitted in any form or by any means, including photocopying, recording or other electronic or mechanical methods, without the prior written permission of the author or publisher, except in the case of brief quotations embodied in critical reviews and certain other noncommercial uses permitted by copyright law.

DISCLAIMER:

The information, situations and persons referred to in this book are based upon actual events and circumstances; though, in some instances, names, locations and other identifying information has been changed to avoid offending or embarrassing the unwary. In this process, some of the people described have become composites, as characteristics of certain individuals are mixed and blended.

The advice given and strategies outlined within this book and associated electronic media may not be suitable for execution by every doctor or medical practice owner. This book is sold with the understanding that the Author and Publisher are not considered to be legal or accounting experts, and the information contained herein is not to be considered as legal or accounting advice. Neither the Author nor Publisher shall be liable for damages arising here from. Citations of websites, books or methods within this book shall not be construed as endorsements of the same unless otherwise explicitly indicated. Further, readers should be aware that the Internet is dynamic and certain references herein to specific websites and technologies may be invalid due to any number of circumstances.

FIRST EDITION December 5, 2019

Copyright © 2019 DigitalGoals, Inc.

All rights reserved.
**ISBN:** 9781671248342

# Contents

*Acknowledgements*

*Prologue*

   The Library Mezzanine

   Bar Napkin Math

   Superbowl Sunday

## PART I: PLAN

### Chapter 1: The Current Environment for Doctors

   The Current Environment for Doctors

   Three Methods to Grow Your Practice

   The Six-Month Lookback

### Chapter 2: Mindset

   No Entry

   Ten Traits We Seek

   Mirror, Mirror

   Of Sorts

### Chapter 3: Who Am I & Why Should You Trust Me?

   Small Time

   Big Time

   Bad Time

   Story Time

### Chapter 4: The Dumpster Dentist

    Matters of Consequence
    Dumpsters and Jail
    Clean Bill of Health

## Chapter 5: Health Care Millionaires
    Cholecystectomies: 97% Off!
    No Business Like Show Business
    Shoot for a $10.8 Million Exit.

## Chapter 6: Get a Coach
    The Gold Standard
    Coaches and Roaches
    Nick, Can You Be My Coach?
    The Importance of Geographic Exclusivity
    Picking a Coach
    Final Word on Coaches

# PART II: BUILD

## Chapter 7: Principles of Digital Scale
    A Ferrari or $200k Cash?
    A Billion Dollar Dentist
    The $12.8 Billion Dollar Doctor
    1968 Was Long Ago?
    No Help?
    Beating the Odds

## Chapter 8: On Internet Marketers
    Here's Jonny!
    Lambo Livin!

    HIPAA Compliant Hosting Violations
    Potential Jail-time for Facebook Violations

**Chapter 9: Real Patient Acquisition**
    Your Web Presence
    Citations: GMBs, NAPs and MAPs
    5 Star Ratings
    A Video is Worth 1.8 Million Words
    Social Media: Mostly Facebook

**Chapter 10: Track Everything**
    The Sole Metric: Top Line Revenue
    Data Collection: 3 Key Methods

## PART III: ACQUISITIONS

**Chapter 11: Growing Via Acquisition**
    Finding Practices to Buy
    Checking Financials
    Of Entities and Taxes
    Letters of Intent
    Your Teammates

## PART IV: EVERYTHING ELSE YOU NEVER WANTED TO KNOW ABOUT INTERNET MARKETING

**Chapter 12: Who Not How**
    Once Upon a Time Near Washington D.C.

Start With Fundamentals

**Chapter 13: How to Setup Your Own Website**

Navigation

Give Them a Reason to Choose Your Practice

Describe Your Services and Service Areas

Reviews and Testimonials Are Important

Make it EASY for Them to Contact You

Is Your Website Mobile-Ready?

**Chapter 14: Uderstanding HOW Search Engines Work**

**Chapter 15: Search Engine Optimization**

How to Conduct Keyword Research

How to Optimize Your Website

How to Build Authority

**Chapter 16: Google Maps Optimization**

How to Establish a Strong NAP

Best Practices to Optimize Your NAP

How to Get Online Reviews

**Chapter 17: Website Conversion Fundamentals**

Example of a Dental Site That is Built to Convert

**Chapter 18: Mobile Optimization**

Hey Siri: Find Me a Doctor!

Text Marketing

Mobile Self Analysis

Spy On Competing Practices

Get Prospective Patients to Call Your Practice

## Chapter 19: Social Media Marketing
When and How to Engage
Notes From the Facebook Front Line

## Chapter 20: Video Marketing
Video Helps with Your Overall SEO Effort
What to do with your video content
Some YouTube Best Practices
What to Send and How Often
Get & Stay Legal with Video Email

## Chapter 21: GoogleAds Profitability
The Google Ads Auction Process
How to setup your PPC Campaign for Success
Mobile PPC Optimization

## Chapter 22: Pay-Per-Lead Programs
PPC vs Pay-Per-Lead (PPL) services

## Chapter 23: Track, Measure AND Quantify
Keyword Tracking
Call Tracking

## Chapter 24: Next Steps
Need More Help?

## Epilogue

## Author's Note

## About The Author

**To Jes, Nicko and Big Mike:**

Thank you for loving me.

Never forget that the foundation of our family's happiness & success is helping other families to be happy & successful.

We all want the same thing.

## ACKNOWLEDGEMENTS

The need for this book is evident. Medical and Dental doctors are brilliant, but not adequately trained in the running of their practices in a profitable manner or the marketing of their services to patients via the Internet. Nor does their extensive education prepare them for the intricacies associated with buying or selling a practice.

It's important to note that DigitalGoals is a family business, and in this way the soul of our business reflects that of the medical and dental practices that we help. Most practices are family businesses.

DigitalGoals isn't some nameless faceless mega-corp situated in far-flung California with thousands of clients. We built this company right in the town that my wife Jes grew up in with the goal of working with the finest family-run medical and dental practices in the country. We actually HELP the families that own these practices to achieve their goals; and, in a lot of cases, we can do what we do in a cost-neutral way that can feel like its "free of charge" to the practice.

I am also indebted to the collective talents of the Executive Masters in Cybersecurity Program at Brown University. Former Executive Director Dr. Alan Usas and my advisor Dr. Jennifer Madden are the two academics who have most closely guided what could or could-not necessarily have been compiled for my Critical Challenge Project (CCP). As a result, this book is very different than the vision I had originally conceived and is perhaps now better.

Professors Linn Friedman and Deborah Hurley deserve recognition for their careful guidance and instruction regarding HIPAA and HITECH as they relate to massive hospitals, assisted care facilities, and most importantly: local medical and dental practices.

Professor Timothy Edgar has my thanks for both his kindness and for the excellence of his thorough instruction regarding law and policy. A little further north of Providence, RI along the cobblestone streets of Cambridge, MA, Harvard's Dr. Christopher Robichaud's past teachings regarding ethics echoed in my ears while writing about matters of moral import.

Finally, to my partners and team members at DigitalGoals: I am grateful for the continued patience and understanding granted by members of our 2016 - 2018 investor cohort: Jon & Jan, Heather & Matt, Andy & Aga, Jimmy, Novella & Bill, Dave and Matt.

It may seem crazy to put forth a map of our business model, but humans like transparency and doctors are no different.

People tend to do business with people that they know, like and trust. I haven't held back much in the writing of this book, so if a reader chooses to engage with us, *then they like us for being us.*

A big part of success in the world is knowing who you are and not trying to pretend you are otherwise. Embracing your destiny, however strange the form, is true freedom.

Thanks to my parents Nick and Betty as well as my two best friends Jes & Andrew for helping me to realize that.

Finally thank you to my sons Nicko and Mikey, without whom I'd never have had the courage to share my experiences in this book and via my podcast: *The Billionaire Whisperer.*

# PROLOGUE

## The Library Mezzanine

Dark, ornate wood & deep crimson carpet adorn the walls and halls in the Harvard Club of New York City (HCNY). It's a formal but social place where alumni can gather and either talk business or cut-loose a bit over a scotch and soda. It is meant to mimic the congenial feel that the members felt as students during their time in Cambridge.

Special Interest Groups (SIGs) abound at the club, some with concentrations as common as chess or specialized real estate investing and others a bit less so, like nude figure sketching. This year I had the somewhat dubious honor of being named the leader of the Poker SIG. While some look askance at a game closely associated with gambling, it's a great way to network with brilliant minds and have a bit of competitive fun. There are quite a few billionaires who play competitively for charity in New York, this fact has made our little group a popular training ground.

For athletically adept members, there are squash courts and a reasonably well-appointed gym; but the primary draw of the club for most members is the use of the dining facilities and bars to socialize and backchannel deals that may eventually be closed in one of the boardrooms upstairs. These beautiful conference rooms are equipped with advanced, motion tracking video conferencing gear that facilitate the attendance of members and stakeholders who cannot be physically present in Midtown.

There are a great many fictional accounts of these wood paneled, cigar-smoke-filled-boardrooms that have played host to meetings where the elite gather to discuss plans to increase their collective wealth and power. I want to assure you that such tales are pure fiction, *for there is no smoking at the Harvard Club.*

I mention HCNY for two reasons:

First, it is the venue where I've chosen to pen this book. Very specifically, the second-level library mezzanine that overlooks the cavernous Harvard Hall. I chose this perch to channel the energy and ethos of the leaders who have graced the space with their brilliance. In years past, the Hall has seen both U.S. Presidents Roosevelt and President John F. Kennedy make their pleas to reason and emotion. In the past few months, the Hall has hosted talks by the brilliant female Chief Investment Officer of Goldman Sachs ISG, Sharmin Mossavar-Rahmani as well as two men whose thoughts I credit much of my own success: billionaires Ray Dalio founder of the world's largest hedge fund, Bridgewater Associates and Eric Schmidt, former CEO and Executive Chairman of Google (and its subsequent incarnation Alphabet).

Second, the Club is a place where my wife Jessica & I invite our clients and their spouses when we all happen to be in Manhattan.

We enjoy with them a private, slow dinner where we discuss our mutual familial and personal ambitions. The privilege of hosting these dinners has taught Jes & I that our clients' hopes, and dreams very much mirror our own.

Here are a few common dreams we share with our clients:

- Healthy, happy and productive children who have been or will be educated at by the most capable educators at the finest institutions of learning on Earth.

- A profession that is rewarding, exciting and lucrative, with work product that is recognized as the standard for excellence in our respective peer group.

- A home that is beautiful, comfortable and large enough to host family and friends for as long as they choose to bless us with their company.

- Security in the form of substantial liquid-assets, or, near-liquid-assets. This liquidity buys-away the unhappiness that accompanies financial worry.

- Travel that is as easy and frequent as it is exotic and exciting.

- A spouse's passion project that could take the form of a non-profit cause, a Pilates studio or a cranky vintage Ferrari.

So, I hope the writing of this book at HCNY will invite many returns in the form of client dinners where we look forward to jointly accomplishing seemingly improbable goals for the future, while holding the understanding that we do actually work to live and do not live to work.

## Bar Napkin Math

I wrote this book in large part because I was tired of seeing doctors being taken advantage of by underhanded-spikey-haired Internet marketers and unscrupulous insurance companies.

We can't work with everyone and thus cannot protect everyone. The math is impossible.

Let's talk about the math: Let's pretend we are at the downstairs bar at HCNY and I flip over the napkin underneath my scotch and I use one of the ever-present crimson-colored-pencils to work a little (easy) math.

Prior to going through this exercise, I'll note that, while the math is simple, its provenance is a bit fuzzy due to the crossing of a number of years and statistical sources. With that in mind, lets agree for the sake of argument that the numbers I present here are reasonably accurate and at least directionally correct.

According to the Kaiser Family Foundation (KFF), as of March 2019, there are 1,005,295 total physicians in the United States, split approximately 48% and 52% primary care to specialists, respectively. Dentists in the United States were reported to be numbered 199,486 as of February 2018 by the American Dental Association (ADA).

One might assume that at most, the audience for our services at DigitalGoals is the sum total of ~1.2 million doctors and dentists practicing in the United States; but that number is far too high for any single company to personally address. So, we only focus on a select set of doctors & dentists who own their own practice, whether that practice be of a medical or dental specialty.

The American Medical Association (AMA) reported in 2017 that approximately 47.1% of physicians owned and operated their practice, compared to the 80% of dentists who are reported to own and operate their practice by the ADA in 2015. So, the functional audience for our services drops to around 633,000.

Out of the 633,000 US based doctor-owner-operators, we have the capacity to work with around 1% of them for an annual Health Insurance Portability and Accountability Act (HIPAA) and Health Information Technology for Economic and Clinical Health Act (HITECH) training and compliance certification.

For these some 6,330 practices we can provide inexpensive and largely automated federal compliance that largely insulates these practices and the personal accumulated wealth of the doctor-owner from expensive HIPAA lawsuits and government fines that could reach into the millions of dollars.

You'll later read in this very book how HIPAA violations and lawsuits have effectively decimated multiple American practices and the doctors' reputation along with his or her life savings. Tragic indeed.

Our training and certification solutions are a form of cheap, effective insurance. A "no-brainer" if you will. It's an easy decision for the doctors, but what they don't see is that their results from training and certification program provide data points that serve as indicators of success to our team at DigitalGoals.

We use this data to score, sort and filter practice invitations for an elite cohort of doctors that we call the "Elite 300 Program." Roughly 10% of the 6,330 practices will report metrics, combined with practice-operational factors that, with our guidance can help them absolutely dominate their respective specialty in their geographical area.

This is not the end of our calculation, for any specialty boutique advisory firm that purports to advise some 6,300 practices is neither boutique nor is it specialty.

Due to the power of the techniques that we employ, we commit to our Elite 300 clients that we will not work with other practices in their geographical area; to do so would be to compete vigorously with ourselves to the ultimate detriment and dissatisfaction of our clients. It is for this reason that we employ strict geographic-exclusivity conflict checks. Since our marketing is conducted on a city-by-city basis, it is not unthinkable that we may supply HIPAA & HITECH training and compliance to two or more practices of similar geography and specialty.

Mr. Nicholas Shawn Chavez

If any or all those practices have the combination of metrics and practice factors that we consider to be reasonable indicators of potential success in the Elite 300 Program, we will invite them to apply to the cohort. Geographic exclusivity is awarded on a first-come-first-served basis and will remain locked until such time that the client discontinues their relationship with DigitalGoals due to merger, acquisition, divestiture or agreement termination.

As of the date of this book's publishing, DigitalGoals has never had a practice cancel a contract. This is rare, so we are proud of it.

Anyway, due to client retention and our rigid geographic exclusivity policy, we cannot service all practices that are interested in our services. This can and has caused some hurt feelings for hopeful doctors and their local practices, especially those who have been invited by us to join, only to be beaten to the punch by a doctor who places a deposit to secure the geography while the other "takes time to think."

We have historically constrained the number of practices that we engage in this program to a total number comfortably south of 500 across all medical and dental specialties. Even toward the upper end of a 500-practice capacity, this still represents less than 0.0008% of the overall doctor-owned practice market in the United States.

The bi-directional loyalty this creates is perhaps outmoded in this, the 21$^{st}$ century; but it has served all parties well enough where DigitalGoals still feels quite comfortable choosing sides with a single doctor per area and playing to win.

Once an agreement is made we sign mutual-non-disclosure clauses with every client. We see no advantage in forewarning your competitors of our plan to extract high-value patients from their practice, siphoning-off high-margin procedures that may very well have been theirs.

Remember, to forewarn your opponent is to forearm them.

## Superbowl Sunday

An interesting story along the lines of non-disclosure, is worth telling, because it contains within it the moment that I decided to write this book.

It happened that we were visiting with a couple in our neighborhood for Superbowl Sunday and a sumptuous dinner. The husband, a former Managing Director for Goldman Sachs and now a portfolio manager for an international fund launched a question: *"You know Nick, I'm not even really sure what it is that you do."*

Interestingly, I've never really had an especially tuned "elevator pitch," despite the seemingly constant professional admonishments to develop one. I usually just tell people that I am an entrepreneur in the health care and financial industries and most folks are content to leave the conversation there.

My neighbor wasn't. He is possessed of the depth of intellect necessary to parse my multiple business models, as well as the connections that could oversubscribe a multi-million-dollar medical or dental practice roll-up-fund in a single phone call. So, I paused and thought of the simplest explanation I could because I'd once heard that long explanations are an indication that a person doesn't really know what he or she is talking about.

**"I help doctors increase the revenue of their practice and then help them leverage the new revenue to buy more practices and get rich."** was the simplest response that my brain could summon.

His eyebrows lifted, "Wow. Nice market!" he exclaimed. I then explained some of the details around our sweet spot of working with doctors to increase their revenue by a target of 300%. "What's the average revenue?" he asked. I replied that our multi-location dental clients are generally bringing in seven-figures in sales per year, averaging around $2.3 million annually and the physicians' practices with whom we seek to work vary wildly by specialty, but again are in the seven-to-low-eight-figure-range annually.

Our host nodded as he chewed his filet. "Good. Good. Don't ever tell anyone about your model. It's a good one." he said as he pointed his steak knife in my direction. I held my hands up in mock-surrender as I laughed. I responded saying that I'd been rolling the idea around in my mind about writing a book about the DigitalGoals model.

Our host was astonished.

"Why in the hell would you do that?!" he sputtered nearly choking on his cabernet. "Don't you think someone will steal the idea? What if someone bigger than you reads the book and decides to use money to muscle you out of the business! *Writing a book is folly."*

I laughed it off and told him he was "probably right" as we enjoyed the rest of the game along with a fine Montecristo cigar and an 18-year-old Macallan.

His scolding sat with me uncomfortably for the balance of the night; but as I brushed my teeth before bed, I resolved to write this book for the following reasons:

1. Doctors help the people that all of us love the most. Why shouldn't they also be rich?

2. Our firm cannot possibly grow to help the top 1% of existing doctor-owned medical and dental practices, (over 6,300 in total in the United States alone).

   While I will not give ALL of our secrets away in this book, the balance of those doctors we cannot personally help DO need some actionable guidelines for success so they don't get scammed by spikey-haired-Internet-marketers or pushed aside by centi-million-dollar Internet marketing warehouses.

3. I'm not really worried about the "competition" in either the Internet marketing realm or the practice acquisition realm, reason being that DigitalGoals has two massive competitors and hundreds of tiny, dinky, irrelevant ones who THINK they can compete with us.

   Let's talk about the big guys first.

   The two large Internet marketing competitors are Scorpion Internet Marketing which did around $254 million in 2018 and Gannett which did roughly $781 million in 2018.

   I know instinctively that they cannot touch us. We are too good at what we do; further, we only work with doctors and dentists.

   Both of our largest competitors claim to specialize, but they serve many thousands of clients from plumbers to attorneys to restaurant chains to large hospitals. When prospective doctors ask us who our competitors are, I never hesitate to mention Scorpion and Gannett.

   I want doctors to price shop us against them because we provide better, more intimate service for a lower price.

I like to say that it's the difference between banking at Wells Fargo and going in and shaking the hand of a bank president that you went to high school with who personally approves your loan. Wells Fargo is a fine bank, but even with its massive capital base and countless branch locations, it's tough to compete when you've got a relationship with a bank president that can make your financial dreams come true right?

The two aforementioned behemoth competitors aside, most other Internet marketers are, by and large, grifters with little formal education and almost no detectible background in technology. Some hold questionable doctorates from long-bankrupted, non-regionally accredited schools, and some are quite proud of their drop-out status.

Either way, we do not see these little entities and their wildly titled "experts" as anything more than a nuisance.

So, all things considered, you now hold the once-verboten book in your hands. I do hope you benefit from it.

The knowledge contained herein should be nearly enough to triple your top line revenue if your practice is making high-six-figures or up to mid-seven-figures in certain markets.

I say "nearly" enough because the knowledge alone is not sufficient. Tripling one's revenue takes discipline, work ethic and some excellent advisors; but, it can be done.

*Here's to folly!*

# PART I: PLAN

*Man is made or unmade by himself.*

*In the armory of thought he forges the weapons by which he destroys himself.*

*He also fashions the tools with which he builds heavenly mansions of Joy, Strength and Peace.*

*By the right choice and true application of thought, man ascends to divine perfection.*

*By the abuse and wrong application of thought, he descends below the level of the beast.*

*Between these two extremes are all the grades of character and man is their maker and master.*

*Of all the beautiful truths pertaining to the soul, none is more gladdening or fruitful of divine providence and confidence than this:*

<u>*Man is the master of thought, the molder of character and the maker and shaper of condition environment and destiny.*</u>

Derived from *As A Man Thinketh* written by James Allen, as told to the author Nicholas Shawn Chavez at the age of 23 by his first outside mentor, Tyger Lucas.

# CHAPTER 1

# THE CURRENT ENVIRONMENT FOR DOCTORS

The famous showman P.T. Barnum had a simple, perhaps crass euphemism that he'd use to describe revenue, he called it *"The Art of Money-Getting."*

I bring up Barnum and his preferred, if somewhat coarse nomenclature for revenue to confront head-on any discomfort that you, as a doctor may have with seeking to be paid significant amounts of money in exchange for your expertise.

You deserve to be wealthy.

## The Current Environment for Doctors

In the 2020's and 2030's health care will continue to change, but whether the industry at-large evolves or continues to devolve remains to be seen. You need to figure out in advance how you are going to play the game, and if you are going to play by some of your own rules or if you are going to let insurance companies call all of the shots.

Even today, some docs might feel a little bit alone in the struggle to care for their patients and provide their family the life they always fantasized about while putting in hard hours in medical or dental school. Some doctors we've talked to run a practice but work side-gigs at urgent care facilities just to make payroll. It's crazy.

With this struggle in mind, I'd like to encourage the following:

## YOU BELONG WITH US

You are a doctor, so it's pretty safe to assume that you were already smart before you picked up this book; but, by reading this book, you are joining a group of knowledge-seeking doctors who have *also chosen to read this book.*

Those other doctors, like you, want to reap massive financial rewards for their skilled-efforts but do not yet understand how to do so.

Myself and the balance of the team at DigitalGoals can help you, but you can also help each other as colleagues in the medical and dental professions. Seek one another out and talk about the methods described in this book. Get better, together.

## THE STATUS QUO IS TERRIBLE

Despite your substantial education and lofty position as a doctor, you are being marginalized by the current ecosystem of corporate medicine / dentistry, large insurance companies, politicians and lobbyists.

You are doing the most important work in the world. You deserve to be paid accordingly. Don't let the corporations win, build a massive practice on your own. Do not get absorbed by the 'borg, instead consider building a practice that is worthy of being called your "legacy."

We can help many practices turn those horrible insurance companies into cash cows for your practice without taking on a single extra patient if you so choose.

## YOU CAN WIN

If there are doctors who have reached deca-millionaire,

centi-millionaire and billionaire status, you can potentially do the same with the right system, advice and funding. Believe in yourself and find someone else who believes in you.

With that foundational understanding laid, I will cover a lot of ground in this book. I generally like to educate through stories; generally, because most humans hate explanations and lectures.

That said, I know that some doctors may only have budgeted enough time to read a single chapter on a plane flight or taxi trip to the airport after attending a conference where we had met.

If that's true for you, I'm sad that you won't get to read some of my sometimes meanderingly-awesome stories; but I get it, time is money.

## Three Methods to Grow Your Practice

Let's get the most important information out of the way right up front: *there are only three methods by which you can grow your practice revenue:*

1. <u>PATIENTS NOW</u> (Get new patients)
2. <u>PATIENTS LATER</u> (Make more money per patient)
3. <u>PATIENTS FOR LIFE</u> (Get a patient to buy repeatedly)

These three methods of growth may seem elementary and intuitively obvious; however, they are worth putting in front of you in black and white. We are going basics-first because, with all due respect, based upon my observations, most doctors are only slightly better at marketing than I am at performing appendectomies[1].

Let's dive in to the three methods:

## PATIENTS NOW: Get New Patients

Getting new patients can only be done in the following ways:

1. Marketing
2. Acquiring another practice

I know some of you are mentally screaming at me "REFERRALS NICK, DUH!", but I caution you that you would not get ANY referrals unless you were somehow marketing yourself either through an alumni association, conferences, word-of-mouth, etc.

And, most prospective patients still check your Google and Facebook reviews AFTER they are referred to you anyway.

*Everything you do is marketing.* From the extra time you spend with a patient to make her feel "heard" to your practice name on the license plate frame of your BMW, to the money that you spend with Google and Facebook to reach the potential patients in your city.

It's all marketing; and we will go through a LOT of marketing information in this book. I will take you step-by-step through the most important aspects of Internet marketing for your practice.

As for acquiring practices, we will cover that later as well.

## PATIENTS LATER: Make More Money Per Patient

Getting an insured patient to pay more for a procedure when the procedure is already coded by insurance is an impossibility; however, for certain physician clients who rely primarily upon insurance, Medicare and Medicaid, we provide a complimentary coding audit to make sure you are billing the insurance companies for all of the work that you are actually doing. It is the easiest way for us to help multiply your practice revenue, and it is ZERO RISK.

If we can't help, you don't pay.

For dentists and other types of physicians who are more reliant upon specialty procedures or perform procedures that are not generally eligible for reimbursement by insurance, Medicare or Medicaid, we will build an Internet marketing program to *find patients in your geographical area who have the wherewithal to pay cash.*

You don't think patients can afford specialty procedures out-of-pocket? Well, it's hard to believe that some consumers will spend $18.9 million on a Bugatti as Dr. Ferdinand Piëch did in early 2019 for his custom one-off automobile.

The crazy thing is, that consumers were so impressed with the car that Bugatti decided to make a production car based upon the Piëch's one-off. The derivative result was the Bugatti "Divo" and is priced much more "reasonably" at $5.8 million.

That's crazy money but is small in comparison to the luxuries I see when I stay in NYC in Battery Park City.

The harbor at Battery Park City plays host to yachts that are often 150 feet long; the owners of these yachts pay upward of $30 million for the yacht on average. The berths alone were sold for $15,000 per foot back in 1989, which means a 150-foot berth would have cost $2.25 million in 1989. To park a boat.

I'm putting these images of multi-million-dollar cars and fancy gleaming white yachts in your mind to illustrate that there are a great many consumers out there who will pay a tidy price to get something that makes them happy or that buys away unhappiness from their lives.

I'm not sure that I'll ever want a yacht or a multi-million-dollar car, but I am not opposed to spending money on my health.

There are a great many wealthy individuals who understand that they cannot enjoy a life of luxury without good health and a youthful appearance. The good news is that there are a LOT of households in the US with a decent amount of disposable income.

In 2018, there were 127.5 million households in the United States; and the top 10% are making $175k per year or more. Since 2014, 100 new billionaires have been minted in the U.S. and there are now over 1,000,000 households in the U.S. with over $5 million in investible assets.

On the low end, that's not Bugatti or yacht money; but I'd be willing to bet some of those assets could be used to buy a desired medical or dental procedure annually if the person so chose to direct his or her discretionary funds in such a way.

Those are the patients we are going after. The top 10% of income earners in the United States, or roughly 12.75 million households.

(Let that HUGE number sink in for a moment. 12.75 MILLION HOUSEHOLDS) That's a mind-boggling number.

Consider this: Gillette Stadium (where the Patriots stomp every other team in the AFC when playing at home) holds 65,878 screaming fans. In order to hold one prospective patient from each 12.75 million well-heeled U.S. household, we'd need 190 stadiums the size of Gillette Stadium.

That's a lot of butts in a lot of seats. We want to put them in your practice's waiting room.

Mr. Nicholas Shawn Chavez

**PATIENTS FOR LIFE: Get a Patient to Buy Repeatedly**

Retention is all about attention.

While many doctors do have goals for revenue, they do not have a system to regularly achieve that revenue, or the tools to implement that system in a reliable, repeatable manner. It appears that their practice is orderly, but their cashflow is anything but. That's a problem.

I was sitting with an OB/GYN last week at one of my favorite Italian restaurants in Denver called Carmine's on Penn, and I was helping he and his wife to understand the basis of the service that we provide to doctors at DigitalGoals. I explained to him that the restaurant in which we sat enjoying our spaghetti carbonara and baked ziti was really not all that different an economic model than his OB/GYN practice.

I asked him what the most expensive thing in the restaurant was.

He knowingly glanced down to the massive diamond ring on his wife's hand and we all laughed. His wife guessed that it might be a 1982 Château Lafite-Rothschild from the formidable wine menu.

In a way, they were both on track. Those are both expensive items, but the most expensive item in any restaurant, *for the restaurant* is an empty table. The same goes for your practice. An open examination room or operatory means that the potential revenue that it could have generated in that time slot is <u>forever lost</u>.

For this reason, we implement one of two strategies:

    1. For our Elite 300 clients, we offer the option of routing

all their new patient calls to an external call center filled with sales professionals who are trained to schedule high value medical and dental appointments.

When these sales professionals are NOT working on inbound calls, they make outbound calls to existing patients to schedule follow-up procedures.

This option seems expensive to docs at first, but it generally replaces the salary of someone that they'd have in-house doing something similar but in a comparatively inefficient manner.

(If you need another example of how this works, try to call a Hilton, Hyatt or Marriott hotel in your city and ask for a reservation. They will almost certainly connect you with their central reservations call center to book your room instead of the front desk at the location you called. Same principle.)

2. For our clients who cannot afford the Elite 300 optional appointment setting service, we implement a CRM software that will automate much of the patient follow-up on behalf of their front office workers.

    This is a far less expensive option and obviously lacks some of the conveniences and efficacy of the fully answered option but is still preferable to losing appointments due to front desk staff that is undertrained in the art of closing sales.

So, there are your three main ways to increase revenue for your practice:

- Patients Now
- Patients Later

• Patients for Life

As you can see, the concept is deceptively simple to grasp and as you might surmise, the trick is in the execution of both the six-month patient lookback/re-code and the practice marketing.

Before we get into the execution, we must fine tune our minds to ensure our efforts are not at odds with our thinking.

## The Six-Month Lookback

Shakespeare, in his play *The Tempest* coined the oft used phase:

*What's past is prologue.*

This is often true and is why banks rely upon credit reports before making a lending decision, and why colleges look at high school transcripts and why medical schools and dental schools look at college transcripts.

Most human's immediate future is destined to look very similar to their immediate past. This is not always the case; however, we can generalize and say that it is true for the majority.

What were your practice's billings vs. collections for the last six-months? Are you happy with them? My guess is that you feel that your practice could improve monetarily, or you wouldn't be reading this book. Do you want your next six months to look like your last six months?

The good news is, past does NOT need to equal prologue.

Where we often start for certain types of practices is a *free, no-obligation* **six-month lookback at your billing, collections and coding.** This requires us to get pretty intimate with your charting, but we do this remotely and it usually only takes 7-10 business days (depending upon how many other practices we are auditing at the time).

Our CPAs and M&A auditors find all of the Electronic Health Record (EHR) coding that your in-house or outsourced medical billing personnel have been missing and then apply them in a legal and ethical manner to get the most from insurance, Medicare and Medicaid.

**Average Patient Revenue Increase (APRI)**

Our average target an additional $50-75 per patient per visit; but the potential for success is far beyond that. Imagine going from $68,000 per month in billings to $119,000 per month over the course of single month; we cannot promise this level of success, but the audit is complimentary, so most doctors look at the consultation as risk-free.

I'm often asked how long it takes to "see results" for the practice and I'm happy to report that implementing the findings in the lookback-audit can be as quick as 48 hours to 21 calendar days, and the associated cash from collections can come through the door between two weeks and six weeks, depending upon the practice's billing cycle and whether or not they need to "wind-down" operations with an outsourced medical billing entity.

**The "Ideal" Practice**

Another frequent question I get is "how do I know my practice will qualify for the free lookback audit?" so here are is what an "ideal" client looks like for the lookback:

- Medical practice
  - Family Practice
  - Wellness
  - Geriatrics
  - Cardiologists
- 20+ patients per day

- 2+ M.D. / D.O. Providers
- $100,000+ in monthly billings
- Either In-House Billing or short-term Outsourced Billing

Do not despair if your practice does not fall within this neat little box, this is just what our "ideal" practice looks like; where we are fairly certain we can make a near-immediate impact to top line and bottom line revenue growth, usually in the tens-of-thousands-of-dollars-per-month arena.

Generally, if your practice is primarily reliant upon insurance, Medicare or Medicaid for reimbursements, we can almost certainly increase your revenue.

We target a 200% increase in revenue for practices who go through our lookback audit and sign up for our Revenue Cycle Management (RCM) services. If a practice also chooses one of our Internet marketing packages, we'd like to see an increase in top line revenue of an additional 100% over 36 months for a total of 300%.

**How Much Does it Cost?**

Ah. Here's the best part: you can choose.

1. If your practice is only interested in acquiring new patients, we are paid a flat fee of up to $12,500 to create new media that will serve as the basis for your online advertisements; then we charge between $3,000 and $7,000 per month depending upon geography, plus whatever your ad budget is (money that goes directly to Google and Facebook).

2. If you are interested in our Revenue Cycle Management, most of the money DigitalGoals charges is based upon your increased practice production plus your Internet marketing fees and ad budget.

We invoice for the RCM service in two ways:

**Billing:** We charge 7% of the collected claim amount with a monthly floor of $7,350. *For this amount you are outsourcing not only your billing, but your accounting as well.*

Some doctors choose to either downsize or reallocate their back-office staff to make this expenditure cost-neutral.

**Success Fee:** We charge 25% of the INCREASED revenue (using the average of the months tallied in the 6-month-lookback audit).

Here's an illustrative hypothetical:

---

## Month Zero: BEFORE RCM

Practice Type: Family Primary Care
Number of Practitioners: 4
Monthly Billing: $120,000
Monthly Collections: $90,000

Outsourced Coding/Billing @ 7% of Collections: $6,300

*Gross Revenue after Billing Expenses: $83,700*

---

## Month 36: AFTER RCM

Practice Type: Family Primary Care
Number of Practitioners: 4
Monthly Billing: $360,000
Monthly Collections: $324,000

Increased Monthly Collections: + $234,000
Outsourced Coding/Billing @ 7% of Collections: $22,680

Mr. Nicholas Shawn Chavez

Success Fee @ 25% of Increased Collections: $58,500
Elite 300 Internet Marketing Fee: $3,000

*Gross Monthly Revenue after DigitalGoals Expenses: $239,820*

---

That's over 156,000 *extra* dollars in your pocket at the end of the month.

**$156,000. Extra. Dollars. In your pocket. In a month$^2$.**

Don't believe me? After your audit, but before you sign our contract, we will put you on the phone with a current doctor client to prove our estimates.

Keep in mind that the aforementioned numbers were hypothetical numbers for a hypothetical practice; but the numbers shown are still not the "top end" of what we've seen our contracted CPAs and coding specialists achieve.

You just need to do three things for RCM:

1. Trust us for a no obligation 6-month revenue lookback
2. Sign up for a 90-day testing period to track results
3. Follow new charting procedure

*Yes. This is legal. Yes. This is ethical.*

We are going after what your practice is LEGALLY ENTITLED TO from the insurance companies. Period.

It seems so basic, so logical; but when you see the excess cash in your practice account during the 90-day test period, it seems nothing short of magical. On the 91$^{st}$ day, we convert the contract to a 36-month term so we can continue to build out positive incremental per-patient revenue.

During those 36 months, for those doctors who really want to throw gas on the fire, the rest of the book talks about how to leverage the profit from the DigitalGoals RCM program along with our Elite 300 Internet Marketing Program to build dynastic wealth for your family through practice growth and acquisitions.

# CHAPTER 2

## Mindset

Interestingly, there is an area of our beach town where one might purchase a fine home with historical significance. This area is referred to as "Doctors' Row", the homes are stately, handsome and spacious. Make no mistake, they are fine houses, but they are not mansions and many of them can be had for less than a million dollars.

They are a reasonable choice for financially comfortable doctors.

But this book is not about becoming a "financially comfortable" doctor. This is a book about becoming a "rich" doctor. Perhaps not *let's-buy-a-new-Rolls-Royce-because-this-one-is-dirty* type of rich doctor, but certainly a level of wealth that moves far beyond "financially comfortable".

Let me explain what I mean with a little bit of context:

As I write this, I am 40 years old and my wife Jes is 34. Jes is particularly fond of a townhouse in New York in a certain part of the West Village that was (over)priced[3] at somewhere in the neighborhood of $10 million[4].

This price tag represents a distant-multiple of the value of our current home; what's more, the carrying costs alone, assuming a paid-off mortgage, were upwards of $10,000 per month.

During our private showing, a rather famous actor barged through the front door and inquired if the townhouse was still for sale. The real estate agent guided him out the door while politely asking him to book an appointment for later in the day (I don't think she knew who he was).

Strangely enough, I knew this actor through my son Nicko, who trained with him in Denver prior to his college days; but, the actor was ushered out the door by the real estate agent before I could say hello. I couldn't immediately locate his number, but I did have his wife's number. I sent her a text that Jes and I were interested in the house and didn't want to start a bidding war with a friendly acquaintance (especially one with his deep pockets).

We ultimately passed on that house for several reasons, but had we not, it would have taken some real financial creativity for us to pull the trigger on it. Why? Because we are "financially comfortable", and our actor-acquaintance from back home could simply write a check for the house and the royalties from his movies, television shows and commercials would probably cover the upkeep cost without him working another day in his life. Is he obscenely rich? No; but his wealth moves beyond the realm of "financially comfortable".

I want his type of wealth for my family.

I want it for yours also.

I've found that doctors can be reluctant to discuss finances. They find it distasteful, rightly thinking that their calling transcends the banalities of money.

Certainly, a medical or dental doctor in the United States is guaranteed to enjoy some modicum of prosperity. Generally, this looks like a five-bedroom house, a few imported cars, and capable educators for their children for the times that they are not vacationing together as a family on the ski slopes or on a beach. All of these comforts are available to any doctor in our fine country, whether that doctor be average, below average or significantly above average.

Some doctors seek this comfort and a slow to average pace. What some of these comfort-seekers don't realize is that by pressing themselves to work hard in an intelligent, guided manner, they could have comfort *and* significant wealth.

With 5 years of focused time, effort and money, one could generate wealth with his or her practice that can be best classified as dynastic or generational[5].

This is a long way of saying that it's quite possible that these first and second chapters may very well be the last chapters you will read of this book. The subsequent content will directly challenge your ego and the fundamental manner in which you think about your profession, your purpose and the world around you.

If you read-on, trust your feelings about your dreams and goals; they are the best indication of your personal truth.

**If you don't want a fantastic amount of money and a storied career in your field, there is simply no reason at all to finish this book.**

## No Entry

In order to be admitted into the Executive Locker Room at a particular private athletic club in Manhattan, one must know where the unmarked door is and submit oneself for a retina scan. Once scanned and authorized, the electronic locks send an audible signal to indicate that access has been granted. In the personal lockers are freshly laundered and pressed gym clothes, a nearby glassed refrigerator holds cooled eucalyptus scented towels and cold bottled water[6].

To some, this Executive Locker Room is the type of expenditure that seems silly, perhaps even shallow. Why all of the pomp and circumstance just to change clothes after lifting heavy things up, putting them back down and running in place for an hour?

Certainly, one must have options, even in an expensive area like Manhattan, to lift heavy things and run in place for free, or at the very least for a reasonable fee, and certainly without the need for James Bond style biometric access control systems.

Of course, those options exist. They aren't for me, and it's not because I'm extra fancy either.

I pay for the admittance process. It gets me in the right mindset. Once the digital locks admit me, it's GAME-ON. I'm there to work and there are professionals there to help me get past obstacles, physical, mental and psychological that are barriers to me LEVELING-UP. Some of what I pay for is the training, sure; but I mostly pay for the exclusivity. Yes, I pay high prices to ensure others are excluded. Specifically, my competitors. You should do the same.

This isn't meant to sound elitist. *It is elitist.*

I like meeting my competitors and KNOWING that they don't have access to the same resources that I do. I want every single advantage I can ethically get in order to build myself into an intellectual and physical weapon that need only be pointed in the direction of a challenge to ensure said challenge is obliterated. I do this for me. I do this for my family. I do this for my clients.

My clients who pay for our top-tier service rarely call me after the 60-90 days or so that it can take to get them set up on the Elite 300 program (outside of scheduled check-ins of course).

Our process just works; it is incredibly difficult to implement, but once it begins to work, it generally continues to work.

Given this, a call from a client is usually about an anomaly, and anomalies demand my immediate focus. I summon all my capability to attack the challenge to help ensure continued client domination in their geography. So, the fees I pay to train at my club at an elite level, ensures I can tap into this mindset in a split second to destroy obstacles.

Whether they know it or not, the doctors in our Elite 300 cohort are possessed of the same capabilities and focus. I can say this with certainty because our team scans for certain character traits before admitting any practice into the Elite 300 program. It is necessary.

How on Earth would our team have even a *remote* chance to accomplish our lofty goal of tripling practice revenue if the doctor heading the practice doesn't have the mindset of a champion?

## Ten Traits We Seek

When we are evaluating a practice for possible invitation into the Elite 300 cohort, we analyze the owner-doctor(s) to see if they are possessed of the following ten-character traits to ensure they can handle the significant demands of the Elite 300 Program:

**Trait #1: Our Doctors Have a Strong Sense of Ethics.**

Cheating to win is behavior that is beneath that of a true champion.

Doctors must be held to the highest standard because they entrusted with the health and happiness of our children, our brothers, sisters, mothers and fathers. Our doctors render only the services that will improve the lives of their patients. Money is a poor substitute for a clean conscience. *Our doctors are Elite.*

**Trait #2: Our Doctors are Decisive.**

Fast-firing instincts are necessary in situations of life and death, sickness and health. Our doctors recognize the need for expert advice, and they action decisions swiftly and with finality upon considering properly sourced advice. *Our doctors are Elite.*

**Trait #3: Our Doctors Thrive on Pressure.**

When faced with a seemingly impossible situation, below-average and average doctors find reasons that it "would never work." Our doctors find a new gear, and get it done. This can be trained, but often, it truly is innate. *Our doctors are Elite.*

**Trait #4: Our Doctors Have a Superior Work Ethic.**

Probably the most important factor we look for, we seek to find doctors who display mental toughness. Your profession sorts for this early: college, medical school, residency, etc. Doctors must have extensive willpower paired with intelligence and a deep well of energy.

Incidentally, we've found that there are two types of doctors:

The first type takes their foot off the gas when they get out of residency into practice; the second type, mashes the gas pedal to the ground to accelerate past their competitors.

The latter squeeze in one more patient per day, they stay up nights seeking answers for yet-unasked questions in their field. They go to conferences and keep up on the latest thinking in their specialty. They do not fatigue even after thousands upon thousands of hours honing their craft. *Our doctors are Elite.*

## Trait #5: Our Doctors are Addicted to Success.

*Our doctors MUST win.*

Winning may look different to different doctors; however, each of our doctors knows what winning looks like to them and they are relentless in pursuing that ultimate vision. *Our doctors are Elite.*

## Trait #6: Our Doctors Welcome Intelligent Advice.

Our doctors are well considered individuals. They do not take advice on blind faith; they request supporting data. When intelligent advice is backed by credible data, and the result of taking the advice appears to be aligned with their ultimate goal; our doctors do not hesitate to execute on the advice. *Our doctors are Elite.*

## Trait #7: Our Doctors Do Not Compete, They Dominate.

Our doctors realize that competition IS a zero-sum-game. A patient rarely sees two doctors in the same specialty. How many dentists does one patient need? How many plastic surgeons? How many cardiologists?

**A patient in your competitor's examination room is one less patient in yours**. If you truly believe that you are *the best*, it is your DUTY to ensure that you are of service to the largest number of high-value patients in your geographic area. *Our doctors are Elite.*

## Trait #8: Our Doctors are Resilient.

With 100% certainty, I can say that we, along with our client-doctors have made and will continue to make occasional mistakes in execution.

Armchair quarterbacking the situation helps no one. We will document, jointly analyze and learn from our mistakes. This is one of the ways successful humans define progress. *Our doctors are Elite.*

### Trait #9: Our Doctors are Pleased, But Never Satisfied.

Records are meant to be broken by champions.

When goals are set and met, one must create new goals to accomplish. For a doctor in his or her 50's or less, the life of the idle rich is only interesting in small doses, for maybe a month at a time. The usefulness of a skilled doctor compares rather favorably to the usefulness of perhaps a hundred ordinary humans.

Even when finances are ample, our doctors compete to win until they choose to retire wealthy and sell their practice for a generous multiple. *Our doctors are Elite.*

### Trait #10: Our Doctors Build Their Own Reality.

Ideals change because circumstances change.

Age, mortality and time wait for no one. We must all close the chapter on our personal productivity at some juncture. This is not the end of monetary income, though the primary assets are now your accumulated funds, your elite practice and your forecastable revenue earned from your finely crafted patient base.

It is your choice to continue to derive funds from the practice as you age or if you'd rather cash out with a lump sum. You must make this decision, no one can or should do it for you. Our doctors build their reality consciously. *Our doctors are Elite.*

## Mirror, Mirror

Some doctors will have seen some or all of these traits within themselves; other doctors will quietly acknowledge that these elite traits do exist, but do not exist inside of them. Fear not! Every single one of these traits can be honed gradually, one must only have a burning desire to improve.

For those that don't have a burning desire to improve, do not despair. There is nothing wrong with average. By definition, being average is the most common trait in the world. It's comfortable and the American people absolutely need average doctors.

*If you are determined to be average, feel free to put this book back on the shelf or return it to whomever presented it to you without guilt and enjoy your abundance of free time.*

## Of Sorts

Now, I hope I've conveyed in these first two chapters that I am not looking to sell anything to anyone. In fact, I have gone to great lengths to include the methodology of some of our most effective Internet Marketing procedures in Part IV of this book. We do not share our proprietary six-month patient lookback / recode strategy, to do so would be to *literally give money away for free*.

I am not in the selling-to-doctors business. I am in the business of sorting elite doctors from average doctors and helping them implement a proprietary process with which we create a practice-revenue-multiplier program. Pretty simple. I don't sell. I sort. Or rather, I let the doctors sort themselves in or out based upon their self-confidence, natural ability and appetite for risk.

This sorting process is the only mechanism I have to protect my and my team members' time.

Soon, you will learn how to protect your time from low value patients as well (but in a kinder and gentler manner than the admittedly abrupt and somewhat coarse process I use). Funny enough, I outline much of our proprietary marketing system in this book; but if I walked up and handed this plan to an average doctor, nothing would happen. They wouldn't read it, or they would read a bit, then claim it's "too hard to execute." Much like a patient who is prescribed "diet and exercise" or "brushing and flossing," some people just won't do the work and *there IS no magic pill to do the hard work in your business or mine.*

So, in effect, the end of this chapter represents your first opportunity to mentally sort yourself and your practice "in" or opt yourself and your practice "out" of the challenging work ahead.

Candidly, even if a doc chooses to opt-out, it won't be the last time they think of me or DigitalGoals. Eventually, they will have to deal with us or our elite doctors (their competitors) in their geography. So, to those average doctors: *enjoy the short break from us should you choose to take one. We'll see you soon enough anyway.*

For the few of you who are still tracking with me and want to begin learning the keys to geographical dominance in your specialty, I promise to stop all the posturing so you can get to know the REAL me so you can figure out for yourself whether I am worth trusting.

## CHAPTER 3

## Who Am I & Why Should You Trust Me?

### Small Time

I grew up on a dirt road in a suburb of Denver, Colorado. My parents both worked for the U.S. Government in the weapons program for the Department of Energy. They were my earliest mentors and friends. They continue to generously give of themselves today and I imagine they will continue to be generous to a fault until they finally pass, hopefully at an age nearing triple digits. (I do happen to know a few good doctors.)

My story isn't about old money though. My parents both grew up in situations that could be described politely as "modest." They shared clothes with their siblings and my mother even sewed some of her own. Education was not particularly encouraged in their households, my father becoming the first college graduate in the history of his family at the age of 44. My mother worked nights to ensure we were well cared for through our childhood. Due in part to her care for us, combined with her heavy work schedule, she never had the time to finish college, despite her considerable brilliance. She instead invested the money into educational resources for her children, including tuition at private elementary and middle schools known for academic excellence.

Due to the self-sacrifice and love of my parents, my younger brother and I had everything we needed and a great majority of what we wanted, but we were not spoiled children. Other than a loan for $20,000 for my first house that I promptly repaid upon the sale of the house and a subsequent $100,000 loan from my father's 401k for a failed real estate venture in my 20's I never received any outsized funding from my parents (sparing the annual Ben Franklin that accompanied most birthday cards).

I paid for my own tuition to Harvard and Brown Universities. Every nickel. My parents purchased for me my Harvard One ring.

I treasure the gift, not because of what it is or even because of the hard work it symbolized. I treasure it because it made them *so happy* to present me with it.

What I have come to find is that everything is relative. The aforementioned loans from my parents could be construed as a king's ransom by some, and a pittance by others; but I wanted to be transparent about it so you'd have an idea of the advantages I grew up with. In my estimation, I'm not sure that my experience meets the bar for a "silver spoon" childhood, but I also don't think it would be a fair characterization if I didn't acknowledge the privilege I did enjoy with a respectful hat-tip to my parents.

Thanks Mom and Dad, you were the first blessing in my life and your love and support continue to be counted as my greatest life-long advantage.

## Big Time

After I transitioned from my private middle school to public high-school, I was placed into the Gifted and Talented program.

I don't think this was the result of a genius-level IQ as much as it likely was attributable to the academics that I was exposed to in private school being far more advanced than those I was eventually presented with in public high school. The public-school administrators plucked me out of some of my regular classes and placed me somewhere that would keep me out of trouble: in the hands of my Autonomous Learning teacher: Mrs. Jolene Kercher.

It worked, kind of.

My newly constructed class schedule enabled me to take a full-time job at an early desktop computer manufacturer called Packard Bell and I found a pretty girl to spend my time away from the office and class with. Senior year of high school, I took a job at IBM making the decision to skip my high school graduation ceremony in favor of an extended summer client engagement for Lucent Technologies in Naperville, Illinois.

By the time I was 21, I had hit a decent stride in consulting and became an executive (perhaps the youngest ever) for a pre-IPO consulting company called Accenture. I was a young father, and, with my international travel schedule, I missed my young son more than words could describe. Being a father to he and his younger brother has been the greatest joy I've experienced in life.

Fast forward several years, consulting for others was lucrative but the economics paled in comparison to the opportunity to start a consulting firm for myself, which I did. From that small firm, my second-mentor and I built a small publicly-traded entity valued at more than $100 million in less than 60 months.

## Bad Time

I sold my shares in the company and I took my money and knocked around a bit, trying my hand at some oil and gas deals[7].

I made an ill-fated run at Hollywood for a while, trying to network into film and music. I made an independent film with my best friend Andrew and co-hosted the Screen Actors Guild party for the Democratic National Convention in Denver in 2008.

I was rudderless in a way but enjoyed the ride with money in the bank. Three mansions, two Ferraris, a Range Rover, a Jaguar and an Aston Martin later the great recession hit, and it absolutely wiped me out. Completely.

That was dumb. Ouch.

I was 29 before I learned that stupidity can be and often is painful. Even then, I still continued to make mistakes.

I mention this because transparency is important to me. I also mention this background because there are a great many individuals who have never had to survive this type of downfall. Give me a battle-scarred warrior any day over a fresh-faced (but enthusiastic!) battle virgin. I want someone who has been through Hell and come out on the other side the better for it.

You should want that too.

Licking my (mostly self-inflicted) wounds, I went back to what I knew: Consulting. Technology. IBM. I began working in verticals that I'd never previously been exposed to, specifically finance, government and healthcare. I found that I was talented at figuring out inefficiencies in the health care information systems used by the Department of Defense and large health care providers such as Siemens and Medtronic. Consulting led in a roundabout way to an engagement with private equity giant Kohlberg Kravis Roberts' (KKR) portfolio companies to advise regarding the technology specifics of two multi-billion-dollar transactions in the medical space.

That's how I accidentally got into the private equity business... but there's an interesting middle-part to my story that I skipped:

Harvard Club, private equity funds and fancy gym memberships aside, I was and am a pretty down-to-earth guy. I prefer pubs to clubs and beer to champagne. My best friends are butchers, security guards, police officers and call center jockeys. A couple made it as doctors and lawyers and still fewer made it into the tech world.

One in particular made it big with Google and that's where this story gets interesting and relevant to you.

## Story Time

George was a hockey star at our high school and a happy, extroverted guy who made everyone around him feel important and wanted.

George and I were introduced by our mutual friend Brenden who chose me as his Homecoming-hazing-target by dressing me up as the Sugarplum Fairy and making me sing "I'm a Little Teapot" at the top of my lungs in a crowded breakfast restaurant after I pushed a penny down a grocery store aisle with my nose[8].

It was all in good fun and we were fast friends after that.

George was a grade ahead of me and left for Canada to play hockey semi-professionally around the same time I left for IBM and Lucent Technologies in Naperville, IL.

Despite our friendship, we'd lost touch after a while as high school pals tend to do.

It wasn't until a great many years later that I'd heard his name again. A mutual friend of ours said: "You might have made some money, but you've got nothing on our old friend George."

What? Really? Huh. I looked him up and found him easily. We caught up over lunch at my second-favorite restaurant, The

Capital Grille.

I asked him to *lay it on me;* I wanted to know the secret to his success.

"Google." he said in between bites of a hearty Delmonico steak. I shrugged blankly. "Man, I'm into Google. I set up websites for these blue-collar guys in the kitchen remodeling space, asbestos remediation, lawn care, plumbing, painters... all of 'em."

I still wasn't really tracking. "You must be setting up a lot of sites to make the kind of money you're making." I replied.

"Well, yeah we have a lot of clients; but that's not it. We make sure that they can close crazy amounts of business by optimizing their sites for the new Google algorithms. We took one guy from being the 28$^{th}$ largest permit-puller in the state of Colorado to the third largest in like five months. He went from less than a dozen employees to almost a hundred. He's in hyper growth mode. It's freakin' crazy."

I blinked. *"That is crazy George."*

"Yeah!' he chuckled... "We did like $40 million last year, not counting ad spend. I know it's not private-equity sized money like you are used to, but we're doing alright." He winked.

Now he had my undivided attention. My mind raced. Even at a modest margin of 10% profit, George and his partner would be taking home millions per year each in cash. Mind still racing, it locked on the work I was doing in private equity for KKR.

"Do you think it would work for health care?" I asked.

"I don't see why it wouldn't. Our biggest competitor is twelve-times our size from a revenue perspective and they optimize big hospitals for Google." he paused, "You thinking about getting into it?"

I nodded in the affirmative.

George's eyes lit up, he smiled and exclaimed:

*"Giddy-up! Let's do this!"*

With George's early guidance, DigitalGoals is now set apart through our commitment to help build the revenue of elite practices by a target of 300% prior to readying them for sale or prepping them to absorb competing practices.

We build cash flow for practices and as we all know: *cash is king.*

Theoretically, a doctor could literally pay for the entire Elite 300 Internet marketing program through implementing the changes recommended in our free six-month Revenue Cycle Management (RCM) lookback audit. So, where's the risk?

Fast forward to today, Google is a gamechanger for doctor-owned-practices in the medical and dental space. So is Facebook. I was in the right place at the right time and through the guidance of an intellectually generous friend, took the inside track early and it has made all the difference.

So, in George's now (in)famous words: *"Giddy-up! Let's do this!"*

## CHAPTER 4

## The Dumpster Dentist

Linn Freedman is a Partner at the esteemed law firm of Robinson+Cole. She and her award-winning practice are the attorneys that doctors call when they've been notified by the U.S. Health and Human Services (HHS) Office of Civil Rights (OCR) to "prepare for an audit" or that they are under "enforcement action."

Either of these federal notices can be scary for a doctor-owned-practice, whether it be medical or dental. What further terrifies the doctors is usually the fact that the audit will extend outward to their business partners, which can include email providers, web hosting providers, phone companies, software vendors, document management companies, accountants and the like.

It's like my traffic-cop friend told me when I asked if he could "pull anyone over anytime he wanted," his response with a smirk and a shrug: *"Well, everyone swerves a little."*

I was very privileged to receive a thorough education in HIPAA from Linn Freedman personally, as she was one of two professors at Brown University for our Privacy and Personal Data Protection module; the other being Professor Deborah Hurley, Fellow of the Institute for Quantitative Social Science at Harvard University.

The individual and collective brain power that these two women have brought to bear at Brown University is absolutely staggering.

They are each brilliance personified.

It is my truest hope is that you meet them proactively, because if you do not want to meet either of them in a reactive professional context. If your circumstance is reactive, it may be because you are staring down the barrel at a multi-million-dollar fine from the U.S. Government or that your practice was the victim in a massive patient privacy breach.

Or, heaven forbid… both.

## Matters of Consequence

We will talk more about HIPAA compliance and the consequences for not complying in a moment, but first let me share an embarrassing personal story with you.

Hedge fund billionaire Ray Dalio and I are alumni of Harvard and there is a real chance that he and I might bump into one another at a function at our club in New York City.

Normally this would be a happy occasion, but I inadvertently irritated him when I imposed on some of his intellectual property (IP). I did so in a way that I thought conferred respect and admiration. The situation was similar to when Elon Musk named his electric car company for Nikola Tesla. Dalio didn't personally tell me so, but when his IP attorneys called me on his behalf, it was impressed upon me that my overture was not only inappropriate but constituted potential grounds for litigation.

Damn.

Not a catastrophic error, but definitely a costly one given our name was already trademarked, branded and registered in several places; also, it was a major faux pas and made me feel pretty dumb given the fact that I truly respect the effort that Dalio has dedicated to writing his thoughts down in the book *Principles:*

*Life and Work.*

I can best underscore my admiration of his book by stating that if I were terminally ill, and knew I would not be around to offer ongoing advice about life and business to my children, but could present them with a single book as a replacement for my personal advice, Dalio's *Principles: Life and Work* would be that book.

Long story short, I promptly transferred title to our IP to Dalio's law firm with a humble apology. They acknowledged the receipt of the IP and the abandonment of the associated trademarks but did not so much as utter a word of thanks. I suppose I didn't really deserve any gratitude, considering I wasted one of my idol's resources and caused him stress.

It took me a bit to realize that I actually owed Dalio gratitude for an object lesson that could have come straight out of his book regarding his principle to *"Weigh second- and third-order consequences."*

From Dalio's *Principles: Life and Work:*

> *"By recognizing the higher-level consequences nature optimizes for, I've come to see that people who overweigh the first-order consequences of their decisions and ignore the effects of second- and subsequent-order consequences rarely reach their goals. This is because first-order consequences often have opposite desirabilities from second-order consequences, resulting in big mistakes in decision making.*
>
> *For example, the first-order consequences of exercise (pain and time spent) are commonly considered undesirable, while the second-order consequences (better health and more attractive appearance) are desirable. Similarly, food that tastes good is often bad for you and vice versa."*

Clearly, I didn't consider the second or third order consequences of infringing on Dalio's IP. Many humans, including medical or dental practice owners make business decisions without considering second or third order consequences.

Most doctors don't know that they are liable for choices that their business partners make and often choose vendors based upon lowest bid or some other trivial convenience.

Let's look at a few examples where doctors didn't think to consider second and third order consequences and as a result lost either money, their reputation or their practice. In some heinous cases, the doctors lost all three. *They lost everything.*

## Dumpsters and Jail

With fines for HIPAA violations reaching as high as $16 million for a single entity, practice owners are paying attention to the details and looking to train and certify their staff to ensure they are not on the wrong side of an audit from Health and Human Services' Office of Civil Rights.

Sometimes, training your staff isn't enough though. You need to make sure your business partners and vendors are trained too. Even if you don't practice anymore. Yes. Really.

Way back in 2011, the Indiana Board of Dentistry permanently revoked Dr. Joseph Beck's dental license for matters related to fraudulent billing and negligence. Two years after the license revocation, Beck was once again in the spotlight after his former patient's dental records, including their x-rays, credit card information, contact information, insurance information and Social Security Numbers were found discarded in a church parking lot dumpster in 2013.

The Indiana Attorney General called the dumpster discovery

"an egregious violation of patient privacy and safety." All told, 63 boxes of records were found in the dumpster of the Olive Branch Christian Church on the south side of Indianapolis. The contents of these boxes amounted to the confidential records of many thousands of patients.

The case settled in 2015 with Beck's signature on a consent judgement for the comparatively small sum of $12,000. The question is, why was Beck on the hook to pay anything at all if he wasn't the one that disposed of the records in the dumpster? A week prior to the discovery of the records in the dumpster, Beck hired a company called *Just the Connection, Inc.* to retrieve and dispose of his patient records. I suppose one could make the argument that the vendor did what they were paid to do, they retrieved the records from somewhere, and disposed of them elsewhere.

The devil, as they say, is in the details.

It is difficult to find information about this case given its age, but one only needs to Google *medical records dumpster* or *dental records dumpster* to see that this case is far from unique; we see examples from Colorado, Connecticut, Georgia, Indiana, Louisiana, Pennsylvania, Texas all on the first page of Google results. It doesn't take a lot of imagination to extrapolate the size of this problem. The worst part? The doctors are on the hook, every time for what seemed like a routine, cost-based business decision.

I won't go into the instances where HIPAA violations have led to the revocation of medical and dental licenses, but there are many. There's no need to examine here the finer points of the doctors and health care workers who were locked up for a misdemeanor HIPAA violation. No sense in tolling the goodwill loss and negative economic impact of the reputational damage done to the practices or organizations associated with these violators. You get it.

You're smart enough to implement a HIPAA + HITECH training and certification solution, especially when it costs around the same amount as the new iPhone you're upgrading to annually.

## Clean Bill of Health

In 2004 for my 25$^{th}$ birthday, I leased my first Ferrari. It was used, and frankly, it was a beautiful disaster. I didn't have it for more than a few months before it developed some pretty major internal engine issues. A standard Pre-Purchase Inspection (PPI) would have uncovered a lot of these issues prior to my acquisition of the car.

I ended up in a major feud with the dealership that sold me the car but the dealer was kind and ultimately accepting a return of the vehicle.

It was stressful; there was a lot of finger pointing and name calling that I could have ultimately avoided by checking the records associated with what I was purchasing and making a better choice.

To be fair to them, I was lucky that they took the Ferrari back. I should have insisted on an inspection to ensure a clean bill of health. A PPI usually costs $800-$1,300. Cheap insurance for a purchase of that nature.

All of this was over a car worth less than $100,000.

What kind of records-check and PPI do you think a potential acquirer of your medical or dental practice will do once we have put the time and effort into it and built a behemoth practice? In the private equity / mergers and acquisitions (M&A) world, we call this "due diligence." You can bet your bottom dollar that they are going to check everything out before writing a 7-8 figure check to you so you can sail off on your shiny white yacht to Cap d'Antibes.

Do you suppose an acquirer might ask to see your HIPAA training program? What if you could proactively present them with several consecutive years of opinion letters from a respected third-party organization attesting to your evident efforts in HIPAA compliance? Do you think that might have a net-positive impact on the purchase price that the acquirer is willing to pay?

We will talk more about the importance of well documented processes in Chapter 17, but suffice it to say that any potential acquirer or intelligent acquisition target will check your HIPAA-associated processes and whether or not you've been certified as a HIPAA compliant practice (and for how many years).

No one wants a HIPAA OCR fine. No one wants a lawsuit.

No one wants a catastrophic engine failure caused by the neglect of a previous owner.

## CHAPTER 5

# Health Care Millionaires

Journalist Luke Darby wrote a short piece for GQ in April 2019 where he aggregates the 2018 compensation for 62 healthcare executives to total $1.1 billion, or an average of $18 million per exec. He contrasts this salary figure with the $88 billion annually that Americans are indebting themselves with annually to afford medical care.

Yes, the American health care system is messed up. We all know it. Doctors know it better than perhaps anyone else. Occasionally, I'll hear a first-hand account from a client or a friend doctor who battles the system on the front line that slams the entire mess into perspective instantly.

### Cholecystectomies: 97% Off!

Some time ago, Jillian, a dear surgeon friend of mine asked me to guess how much she was paid to remove a gallbladder. My monetary guess was WAY, WAY OFF; she then broke down the process pretty simply:

> "The average cost to the patient in the United States is somewhere between $8,000 and $32,000. But what we collect is an entirely different story!
>
> Generally, the clients do not pay us directly. They may have an out-of-pocket insurance deductible, but that is where the client-pay portion of the insurance procedure usually stops.
>
> We then negotiate with the insurance companies for the

actual collectable balance. Let's use the most commonly acknowledged figure of $24,000 as the cost for laparoscopic surgery; the surgeon usually gets $759 to $900.

To add insult to injury, it is not uncommon to wait a month or more to collect that money from the insurance company."

This particular friend went on to mention that she exited her general surgery practice which had a healthy ~1,000-member patient base to take a general surgery position at a hospital. This part of the conversation I could understand a bit better, because it's all about EBIDTA and multipliers, or so I thought. When I inquired what she sold the business for, I received a blank stare in response. "Well, you really can't sell that kind of practice," she said, "who would buy it?" she inquired.

Her statement hit me like a punch in the gut.

She simply wrote a letter to her patients referring them to another practice in the area that was run by a doctor that she trusted. The goodwill, patient receivables and transferrable patient base could likely have been monetized with sound advice and a little focused effort.

The reason that these seemingly "worthless" health care practices can be monetized is rooted in simple economics: the exiting physician can demand a price weighted against the cost and time necessary to start a practice in their geography. Accumulating a patient base of 1,000 could and likely would take several years.

Additionally, the profitability of any newly established practice is not guaranteed, due to unknown personnel and undocumented and unproven processes. Even a process that is grossing a substantial top-line and losing money every year has a value to the market. We have a name for businesses like that in private equity, they are called "turnarounds."

We will talk more about practice valuations and goodwill in Part III.

I became more and more fascinated by what seemed like a common choice among doctors to simply "shut" their practices and refer their patients to another doctor. As I thought about the historic advertising and marketing costs that went into acquiring those patients, I thought to myself: *"WOW! What a gift to the doctor receiving the referral!"* I also cringed at the thought that I have access to the acquisition price paid for nearly every single medical and dental practice going back to 2002 and could have given her an approximate idea of what her practice was worth in the time span of a phone call.

Since that conversation, my surgeon friend and I have had many conversations; some of which she claimed were helpful to her in pivoting her practice to a fee-for-service aesthetics practice.

No more insurance. Cash and credit only.

She zealously guards her time and will not take a client for less than the several-hundred-dollar-per-hour fee that she charges.

Dr. Jillian is brilliant and seems much happier with her new fee-for-service practice, but I can't help but wonder if she's curious about how much money she left on the table. I'm not going to ask.

## No Business Like Show Business

Some say that CEO's are highly paid because they must make tough decisions daily.

I couldn't agree more actually.

One particular health care CEO I worked with had to make a tough decision as to what to drive to the office every day. Some days he drove his Lamborghini Huracán, or his Aston Martin DB11; however, neither of those would do on especially sunny days when he preferred his McLaren 650S with a retractable hardtop for open-air motoring.

Snow days demanded use of his supercharged Range Rover.

This particular CEO attained an undergraduate degree from an institution that I'd never heard of before and would be hard-pressed to find on a map. Note that I am happy for his success and have always found him to be a fair and admittedly likeable man; but, I find the economic disparity between an individual like him and a doctor who has completed a full eight years of higher education, plus a 2-7 year residency and is charged with actively saving human life daily to be a bit, well... unbalanced.

The disparity between health care company CEO pay and the pay of an average doctor, dentist or surgeon is pretty striking. Let's mark an average physician's pay in the United States around $200,000 and the pay of an average dentist slightly less at around $175,000. These highly intelligent, extensively educated individuals are earning around *one-percent* of what a top healthcare CEO earns annually, according to Darby's GQ article.

Seems a bit backward doesn't it?

Let's think for a moment about the way show business works. Everyone has a favorite actor or actress, and everyone has a different opinion of who is good and who isn't, so I'll just pick someone who I think is indefatigably awesome: *Sir Anthony Hopkins.*

Even if you haven't seen his hits like *Silence of the Lambs, Hannibal* or *Meet Joe Black,* I'd ask that you take it on face value that he's a good actor as his fee per film is ~$20 million.

Not a bad payday, but he doesn't keep all of it; Hopkins is represented presently by what is considered to be one of the top three talent agencies in the world: Creative Artists Agency (CAA). CAA takes a fee of 10% from Hopkins' earnings per film, effectively reducing his earnings by $2 million.

This seems okay right? CAA effectively brought Hopkins a customer and landed him a deal, so a 10% fee feels like fair compensation for the agency bringing the film studio to the table and getting them to agree to the actor's terms.

We aren't done yet: often actors have managers who take another 15% and an entertainment attorney that takes around 5%; so, 30% of the top line revenue is gone, but that is the "cost of doing business."

We all have those costs in our business, and even with those big slices out of the pie, Sir Anthony Hopkins still enjoys a 70% margin on his acting services.

So why in the medical and dental fields is the business so different? Why does a procedure that costs $24,000 pay as little as $759 to the highly educated professional that did all of the work?

I guess it's because health care CEOs seem to get paid more than Hollywood agents do.

## Shoot for a $10.8 Million Exit.

Everyone has their number. The number that is etched in their mind that will provide them whatever the term "financial freedom" has come to mean for them personally. For many working-class folks, that number is and has been $1 million. We talk a lot about this number on *The Billionaire Whisperer* podcast.

Anyway, as we've discussed, most physicians and dentists can make more than $150,000 in almost any city in the United States. There are a great many more who make upwards of $400,000 or $500,000 per year.

No one knows better than I do that $300,000 to $600,000 a year is a comfortable income but brings along with it a disgustingly high tax bracket and a great many personal demands from family, friends and others who think you are already *utterly wealthy*. (you aren't.)

It's not unheard of for a doctor who is making $400,000 per year to live in a multi-million-dollar home, in fact, I'd assert it's quite common based upon conversations that I've had with friends and clients.

We could argue about whether or not that level of spending equates to self-confidence or over-confidence; but I am not interested in passing judgement. I am only interested in helping doctors to be in a position to *write a check* for a multi-million-dollar house and not worry about a mortgage ever again.

One of my early business mentors, Rob, takes an annual staycation with his wife at the stunningly beautiful Broadmoor Hotel in Colorado Springs every November. This hotel is only about an hour away from his primary home, but it's a world away from their day-to-day responsibilities. The purpose of this trip is to analyze the goals that they'd set for the year and their progress toward accomplishing them. This conscious habit of taking a step back, assessing their business and personal goals has played a major part in generating tens-of-millions-of-dollars in the decade-and-a-half that I've known he and his lovely wife (who, incidentally, is as instrumental in Rob's business as Rob is.)

I know this for a fact because Rob helped grow my net worth to deca-millionaire status when I was in my mid 20's. He and my other early 20's mentor, Tyger (as well as my fine parents) taught me much of what I needed to know about building certainty into my mindset.

The takeaway? Write your big number down, look at it every day.

Meditate upon it. Pray about it. Think about your big number and laugh for joy. Think about your big number and cry happy tears. Think about your big number and be grateful for having that large amount of money enroute to you.

Admittedly, there was a time when I thought that this "Law of Attraction" stuff sounded rather hocus pocus. I always thought that I was "too smart" to be tricked into believing something as flimsy and non-scientific as that. It seems to work though. You'll just have to learn that for yourself. If you are a religious person, you'll recognize that the daily practice is not terribly different than one's daily devotional and prayer.

Do this: go somewhere quiet and write down on a clean sheet of paper a dollar figure, something in the single digit millions. It should look like this:

---

$3,000,000

*Good. Now take the $3,000,000 number and divide it by 12.*

$3,000,000 / 12 = $250,000

*Okay, now take the $3,000,000 number and multiply it by 1.8.*

$3,000,000 * 1.8 = $5,400,000

*Finally, take the product of that equation $5,400,000 and multiply it by 2.*

$5,400,000 * 2 = $10,800,000

*Nice. You're done.*

---

You've just set your practice goals. Let's walk through it. The $3,000,000 figure is what your annual top-line revenue will be. The $250,000 figure is the average monthly revenue you will need to achieve your top-line (gross) revenue. With me so far?

The 1.8 multiplier is what I've seen as the average acquisition multiplier in the market for a well-run practice.

Multiplying the product of the acquisition multiplier by a factor of two is what can happen when a target for acquisition shows rapid, non-linear growth and has documented the processes around that growth for replication and scale.

Translated into simple terms, we need to get whatever your top line revenue number is NOW to at least a $250,000 monthly run rate (MRR) and $3 million annual run rate (ARR) for us to have a shot at an exit of $5 million+. If we choose to work together and you follow the recommendations, and the M&A climate is favorable it's not unimaginable that your exit could exceed $10 million[9].

But we are getting ahead of ourselves. First, we need to pump up those rookie MRR numbers that you are doing to *at least $250k*.

If you're already at $250k MRR, great, read on and take the advice to throw a little jet fuel on the fire.

# CHAPTER 6

## Get a Coach

Can you think of a professional sport that doesn't have a coach? I can't.

Sure, we all see NBA, NFL, NHL, MLS and MLB coaches featured prominently with furrowed brows just outside of the field of play calling shots and motivating their teams to win championships. Teams have coaches, many of them are as famous or more famous than the players.

What about the coaches of superstars in sports that are more focused on the performance of a single individual? Can you name the coach who helped either Venus or Serena Williams perfect their backhands or monster serves? How about Tiger Woods' swing coach? Whose words of encouragement swim around Michael Phelps' head at night? What is the name of the coach that took Floyd "Money" Mayweather's boxing to a perfect 50-0 record with 27 knockouts in the boxing ring?

I literally couldn't name a single one of those coaches without looking them up, and yet their protégés are the best in the world in their respective fields. The moral of the story is, the best performers in the world have coaches. Will your ego allow you to admit that you need one too?

Just make sure you pick the right one.

### The Gold Standard

In my opinion, the finest coach in the world was a man named

# RICH DOCS

Bill.

While your mind may have raced to Bill Belichick, the head coach of the NFL's New England Patriots and winner of six NFL Championships, that is not the Bill I am talking about *(even though he is my favorite NFL coach and leads my favorite NFL team GO PATS!)*

The man I am talking about was the former head football coach for the Columbia University Lions, and under his leadership, the Lions won only 12 out of 64 total games in five years.

You're probably thinking: *"Wait. What?"*

Yes, Bill Campbell had a winning percentage of 18.75%. He is not a household name and I *still* consider him to be the best coach who has ever lived.

So did Steve Jobs the late co-founder of Apple. If you were to ask Google founders Sergey Brin and Larry Page, I'd bet my last dollar that they would tell you that they considered Bill Campbell to be the best coach in the world also. John Doerr, arguably the most successful venture capitalist of all time leaned heavily on Bill Campbell for advice, and actively referred Bill to young entrepreneurs in Silicon Valley to form a mentor-mentee relationship.

One of those referrals John made was to the former CEO of a company called Novell Networks, who had departed to work with Google when it was still a startup with less than a couple of hundred employees, this referral was a brilliant executive named Eric Schmidt.

By Eric's own admission, he was already well known and considered to be "bright" by Silicon Valley standards (which puts him squarely in the category of "flipping brilliant" anywhere else in the world) and he wasn't sure that he needed a coach at all. He was actually a bit taken aback by John's suggestion which he admits dinged his ego a bit.

That was in 2001. Fast-forward 10 years to 2011, Eric had been the Chairman of Google for a decade and Bill coached him, and the founders Sergey and Larry through an initial public offering (IPO) of their stock as well as countless product and personnel challenges.

Once, Eric was asked to "step down" as Chairman and thought that he might quit Google altogether. Not to mention the massively negative impact this would have had on Eric's eventual personal net worth (which as of 2019 is an astounding $13.9 billion), he would not have enjoyed the balance of the challenges and accomplishments that he experienced at Google until he finally stepped away from the company in every capacity in January of 2018.

Every Sunday, Bill Campbell would take a long walk with Steve Jobs. Other than his wife Laurene, Steve considered Bill to be his best friend and confidant. In 1985 when Steve Jobs was unceremoniously fired from his own company, Apple, Bill was one of the only voices on the Apple Board that stood up for him and attempted to reason with the board that Steve was just "too talented" to lose entirely. I won't belabor the balance of the Apple story since there is a very good chance you either purchased this book or are ingesting the contents of this book via an Apple device.

The really silly-amazing twist is when you realize that Bill Campbell was advising both Apple and Google simultaneously. iOS and Android: Patents, attorneys, injunctions, lawsuits, demand letters, hundreds of billions of dollars. Both the executive suite at Apple and the executive suite at Google relied on Bill Campbell utterly to get them through the all-out-war that they waged with one another over mobile operating systems.

The result?

Google and Apple together now own nearly 98% of the mobile operating system market with some 3.3 billion devices split between them. So, who won? Well, both companies won because they both had the same amazing coach: Bill Campbell and as a result, the founders don't look at the price-side of the menu when they take their families to Red Lobster.

In April 2019, former Google & Alphabet Executive Chairman Eric Schmidt came to Harvard Club New York to discuss the release of the book *Trillion Dollar Coach* that Eric wrote with long-time-Google co-workers Jonathan Rosenberg and Alan Eagle.

The trio were kind enough to have a chat with HCNY members and sign a few books for us. In the book, they offer contextual examples of Bill Campbells' wisdom and grace for those who are looking to either perform as a coach or seek out a coach. I bought a copy and Alan happily signed it; Jonathan signed it less eagerly mentioning that Eric "does not like to sign books." This appeared to be true, as Eric was inching toward the door and finally called out to his two assistants that it was "time to go" before hopping into the back a chauffeured silver 2019 Mercedes Benz S450 4matic and speeding away.

Still, I was able to ask the panel of three a question about a well-known former Google employee that Eric answered in a diplomatic but comprehensive way. I sent Jonathan a photo that I'd taken of him alongside Eric and Alan to which he promptly replied with an email expressing his gratitude. Three wealthy men, all class acts.

After having devoured their book *Trillion Dollar Coach* within 24 hours of meeting them, I can heartily recommend that you buy and consume the book as well.

For those of you who lack the opportunity to read the book immediately or the time to read it thoroughly, I'll share five principles (of 36) sourced directly from the *Trillion Dollar Coach* book[10] that are most relevant to my opinions about coaching doctors through DigitalGoals:

---

### 1. Only Coach the Coachable:

*The traits that make a person coachable include honesty and humility, the willingness to persevere and work hard, and a constant openness to learning.*

### 2. No Gap Between Statements and Fact:

*Be relentlessly honest and candid, couple negative feedback with caring, give feedback as soon as possible, and if the feedback is negative, deliver it privately.*

### 3. Don't Stick It in Their Ear

*Don't tell people what to do; offer stories and help guide them to the best decisions for them.*

### 4. Be the Evangelist for Courage

*Believe in people more than they believe in themselves, and push them to be more courageous.*

### 5. Love the Founders

*Hold a special reverence for -and protect- the people with the most vision and passion for the company.*

---

Finally, allow me to share an insight from the book that the authors pulled from a 2001 paper by Fiona Lee and Larissa Z. Tiedens that will underscore the reason why a brilliant person needs a coach:

> *"In fact, it is often the highest-performing people who feel the most alone. They usually have more interdependent relationships but feel more independent and separate from others.*
>
> *Their powerful egos and confidence help drive their success but may be paired with insecurities and uncertainty."*

Wow. When I read that, it hit me like a lightning bolt. If it didn't hit you like that, re-read it. Schmidt et al. go on to quote Lee & Tiedens who note that *"power creates a subjective sense of separation and distinctiveness from others."*

I can imagine that you, dear doctor, in all of your years preparing for your career of service to your fellow human, or in the rendering of said service, have felt totally and utterly alone at some point.

You don't have to feel alone.

Find a coach you can bounce ideas off of, one that will care enough about you to occasionally pierce your ego if necessary, one that can pick you up off of the field of battle, arm you with courage and push you back into the fray with the full knowledge that someone has your back and is watching, cheering and strategizing for your win.

## Coaches and Roaches

When I was consulting for the U.S. Department of Defense, I worked with a retired U.S. Army Lt. Colonel who, when asked whether or not I should include certain negative information in a briefing, responded to me "Well, you don't have to Nick; but, you can only lose your integrity once."

Ouch. Long wince.

"Roger that Col." I replied.

I inserted the information in question and dealt with the inevitable consequence of discussing the specifics of the unpleasantries with the client and the military contractor in question.

Integrity is essential to a long and happy career, we all instinctively know this; however, for a great many people in the coaching business, their integrity has a price and they sell it every chance they get.

I do not consider myself to be a "coach" in the strict business-sense of the word, simply because one cannot "buy" my time as a "coach."

Certainly, there is a major aspect of the services that DigitalGoals delivers to our Elite 300 clients that is, definitively, "coaching," but it is coaching in the broader context of execution of specific tactics and strategies to attain a stated goal.

In its most pure form, what we provide is management consulting that should, if properly executed in a fair market, eventually result in a substantial lower to modest lower-mid-market private equity or M&A transaction.

Of course, something as simple as finding a coach is not simple at all.

The primary issue that many doctors find with hiring a coach is that there are just so many charlatans out there, hocking their "expertise" and "proprietary systems." Often these "coaches" are hired with an initial payment of a few thousand dollars to have "access" to their proprietary system, which is nothing more than a few PDF documents and a private Facebook group.

Fine, we've all been swindled in petty ways for a couple hundred or a couple thousand dollars; I'm not too proud to admit that I have fallen for some of that same drivel. It was embarrassing for me at the time and I knew I'd been duped as soon as I sent the wire transfer; perhaps you've fallen for something similar?

Let's get back to coaching and what is probably the most egregious example that I can think of in the medical and dental industry today:

There is a doctor who coaches fellow doctors, more than a few thousand worldwide in his specialty. He charges a fee for coaching and he charges an admission fee for his own personal events that generally occur at the same time and place as the national convention of these types of specialists.

He will identify a partner of sorts who has a product to sell, and in at least one instance I know of, the product being sold can range between $20,000 and $30,000. This doctor might take a 25% commission from the partner who sold the product, plus 10% of any fees generated from his students thereafter. So, that's somewhere between $4,000 to $7,500 he is making upfront PER referred doctor, and an additional $1,000-2,000 per month.

*Not bad money if you have the stomach to sell out your coaching clients, I guess.*

Now, I don't have a problem with people making money and I am also not opposed to paying referral fees to doctors or any other credible source of referrals so long as it is legal and ethical to do so.

## Mr. Nicholas Shawn Chavez

I want people to be successful and I am not a greedy person; however, I do have a problem when a coach sells out his or her students for *undisclosed profit.* That's right, it seems that this doctor-coach's students didn't seem to understand that he was pocketing these massive referral fees from the partner he brought in to speak at his private event.

So, let's break this down. This "coach" got a fee:

1. When a doctor joined his "coaching program" to learn his "proprietary system"
2. When a doctor was upsold into a "mastermind" of his peers
3. When a doctor attended the "private coaching event" instead of the national convention
4. When a doctor took his advice to buy Internet marketing services that his colleague was selling as a "referral fee"

A conservative estimate puts the number of doctors that this "coach" referred to his Internet marketing "partner" at 4-6 dozen.

So, let's do more quick math:

*Conservative Estimate of Referral Fees*

*48 Doctors * $4,000 initial referral fee = $192,000 (up-front referral fees)*

*48 Doctors * $1,000 monthly = $48,000 (monthly-recurring referral fees)*

*Moderate Estimate of Referral Fees*

*60 Doctors * $4,250 initial referral fee = $255,000 (up-front referral fees)*

60 Doctors * $1,500 monthly = $90,000 (monthly-recurring referral fees)

*Aggressive Estimate of Referral Fees*

72 Doctors * $4,750 initial referral fee = $342,000 (up-front referral fees)

72 Doctors * $2,000 monthly = $144,000 (monthly-recurring referral fees)

From my understanding, the numbers are closer to the "Aggressive" estimate than they are to the "Conservative" estimate.

*I could have done a currency conversion to see what if the USD equivalent was more or less than 31 pieces of silver paid per doctor, but who has that kind of time?*

Anyway, this type of structure begs the question, who is this "coaching" relationship designed to help? The student / doctor or the coach himself? Also, before you ask, I am not going to mention the name of this "coach" doctor for a couple of different reasons, not least of all is the litigious nature of our fine country.

His "partner" was a spikey haired Internet marketer. I know this particular spikey haired Internet marketer's playbook pretty well because I know who he outsources all of his work to (and they aren't very good.)

This means that our Elite 300 Program clients should be able to outmaneuver his clients pretty consistently in their respective geographies should they ever go head-to-head.

*Cruel?* Nah. *Competitive as hell?* Yep.

Knowing the other guy's playbook isn't a Bill Campbell move.

It's a Bill Bellichick move (GO PATS!). I want our doctors to dominate this coach's doctors in every way, including market share. Ultimately, I'd like for our docs to buy out his docs' practices for pennies on the dollar because we've absolutely decimated them in a particular geographical market.

Crazy enough, the money paid for referrals is not even the worst part. The sad fact of the matter is that the referrals this doctor made to his coaching students may ultimately expose them to HIPAA fines and potential jail time due to the spikey haired Internet marketer's Facebook advertising methodology.

We will learn more about this perilous situation in Chapter 8.

## Nick, Can You Be My Coach?

Dang. I'd love to be. Coaching is my favorite thing in the world and that is the honest-to-goodness truth.

However, as mentioned previously, we've made a conscious decision to keep DigitalGoals relatively small (i.e. not grow beyond roughly 10% the size of our largest competitors) with the capacity to serve only a few hundred clients in a boutique model.

My overwhelming desire to help doctors paired with my lack of available time is a big driver for the writing of this book. I don't enjoy seeing doctors get ripped off by every insurance company and spikey haired Internet marketing grifter that thinks doctors are "rich."

I know that the vast majority of you are comfortable, but a pretty long way from being truly "rich." There's a big difference, and I do hope that you get to experience being *truly rich* someday, which in my estimation is having at least $10 million in liquid or near liquid assets on top of your primary residence and other real estate. The interest and dividends paid from this amount alone is 2.5x what the average doctor makes in the U.S. annually. You can hear a little more about my thoughts about wealth on *The Billionaire Whisperer* podcast.

Through *The Billionaire Whisperer*, I coach a great many people. I even offer to coach some of them personally for around $30,000 per year. As an Elite 300 practice, you get all of this coaching essentially "free" as it's included in the program.

Pretty sweet huh?

Interestingly, the great Bill Campbell, famed Silicon Valley business coach didn't charge his clients for his coaching time either. They would leave whatever palatial office they had at Apple, Google or Facebook and drive over to Bill's little office and have a powwow with him after hugging his secretary hello; they received no invoice for this service. It was just part of what they automatically got when Bill was on their side of the ball. All-inclusive. Morning, noon or night. If you have an issue, they called Bill's cell.

No one abused the privilege because they knew it WAS a privilege, so they were selective about which problems to bring to Bill's attention. No need to swat at a fly with a sledgehammer.

It's the same with DigitalGoals' Elite 300 cohort. If a doctor has a question, he or she can ring my personal mobile phone directly without any need for an appointment. I might not have the ability to answer immediately, but I always return my clients' calls quickly, especially if they are urgent. It's the right thing to do.

## The Importance of Geographic Exclusivity

Beyond capacity to serve a great number of clients in this personal manner, I constrain the number of doctors I personally advise based upon geography. This is due to a concept that all undergraduates learn when earning their undergraduate degree at Harvard University: I am speaking about the concept of *moral hazard*.

Taught in a class that meets Harvard's *undergraduate ethics requirement,* moral hazard essentially describes a situation wherein someone has an incentive to take risk without taking responsibility.

A good example of moral hazard was shown in the government bailouts of the banks in The Great Recession back in the late aughts. The U.S. Government approved $700 billion to bailout banks that were "too big to fail." This taught bankers that they could make increasingly risky bets with very little negative economic consequence to their bank or their personal pay package. Risky deals usually pay better, so why not go for the upside since the downside risk is borne by someone else? That's moral hazard and it sucks, especially if you happen to be on the receiving end.

Now let's re-center on DigitalGoals' business of advising doctors. What do you think might happen if we were to accept into the Elite 300 cohort two dentists in the same small suburb of Denver?

Certainly, we could advise them both to "dominate" their market and instruct them how they could leverage certain organic and paid Internet strategies to acquire substantially ALL of the dental market share in the small city of Glendale. Initially, neither dentist would know that we were helping another dentist in the city, but eventually they might notice two trends:

> 1. The price of paid Google and Facebook ads for keywords associated with "Glendale Dentist" would be increasing,

making it more expensive for them to acquire market share.
2. They might realistically be losing as many patients as they gain, assuming that DigitalGoals advised both doctors to extract patients from other nearby practices using certain strategies (we do).

Ultimately, neither practice would enjoy the success that they could have experienced if DigitalGoals took the ethical stance to limit the number of clients in a certain specialty within a geographical area to ONE practice; but DigitalGoals might have theoretically collected 2x the revenue it could have charged to represent a single practice by representing two. That's moral hazard.

Most "coaches" don't care about moral hazard.

I do.

That's why I don't generally take personal coaching clients. That's why the only clients that I coach are Elite 300 clients of DigitalGoals, and are segmented by geography and medical practice type for three reasons:

1. To ensure the doctors are not competing with one another
2. To ensure they can target ANY local practice for eventual acquisition
3. To ensure they are getting the best return on investment (ROI) possible on marketing dollars spent

It's worth noting that practices who do not hire DigitalGoals for Internet Marketing services and only choose to avail themselves of our risk-free six-month patient lookback / coding product to increase top line revenue for existing patients are NOT granted geographic exclusivity because we are not bidding for keywords to attract new patients and therefore are not entering into a situation where the potential for moral-hazard exists.

## Picking a Coach

Have you ever seen one of those quasi-inspirational Facebook or Twitter posts by some soft-headed motivational "guru" that espouses some sentiment like: *"You have as many hours in a day as Oprah does."*

*Sigh. <insert eye roll here.>*

First, yes. Right; as humans we all experience time in a suspiciously similar linear manner that was quantified long ago into seconds, minutes, hours and days. Beyond this similarity, the idea that "you have the same hours in a day at your disposal that Oprah does" is almost infuriatingly stupid. Way back in 2012, Oprah had 12,554 employees, which means that she could personally command 301,296 hours in any given day... not including her own 24 hours.

How many people do you think that Oprah has time to personally coach? In all likelihood, the answer is zero. In reality, she probably coaches a few, close, personal friends or mentees; preferring to extoll her knowledge and life-strategies via her talk show which reaches millions of individuals simultaneously via broadcast and cable television.

This is a lesson in economics. Persons who are able to deliver high value to the market will always be in higher demand than those who do not or cannot.

Certainly, one could walk into a Walmart and find some employee and convince that person that you were worthy of his or her time as a mentee. Walking into Walmart headquarters in Bentonville, Arkansas and requesting the CEO of Walmart to spend his time mentoring you would undoubtedly have a very different outcome.

As such, most high value individuals, whether they consider themselves to be a "coach" or not, will have a set of criteria that they use to identify strong potential mentees that they can advise and help evolve from good to great.

Now you can't always tell how successful a coach is by how unavailable he or she may be to persons on the outside-looking-in, but an intractable schedule *can sometimes* be relied upon as a decent indicator of success.

Microsoft co-founder Bill Gates is going to have a different set of criteria for taking on a student who needed some coaching in the programming of systems than would a high-school computer science teacher. The likely commonality between Mr. Gates and a high-school CS teacher is that both will likely want to know what you accomplished with your last coach. This is a great way for them to quickly determine whether or not their time will be well spent in a coaching relationship with an aspiring mentee.

Here are five questions that you should be prepared to ask your coach to see if the relationship fit would be a good one. I'll add my answers to these questions to you can assess whether or not the answers you get from your prospective coach align with mine (whether or not mine are any good or not is subjective; but feel free to use them as a reference nonetheless):

- **What drives you to want to be a coach in the health care industry?**

    I enjoy helping people. If I can be helpful to a doctor to help thousands of people with their gift, then it applies a very strong multiplier effect on my abilities and efforts. One of my early friends & mentors (Jon Biel) said that *"people will never forget you if you help them in one of three areas: health, wealth or their children."*

Health care hits all three.

- **What experience do you have in health care finance and technology?**

I have been instrumental in the completion of a handful of multi-billion-dollar health care transactions in the private equity / M&A market. I've consulted on health care technology matters for multiple Fortune 500 health care companies as well as the United States Department of Defense. I also attended Brown University to earn a master's degree in Cybersecurity.

- **How do you select your mentees or clients?**

Our company provides RCM audits and Internet marketing services to medical and dental practices. Certain practices who participate are invited to apply to participate in our Elite 300 Program.

The leaders of those practices have a personal relationship with me, I do not charge them extra for my coaching services.

- **How are you compensated?**

It depends upon the doctor and their practice, and whether they are interested in generating revenue from their existing clients or would like to simply focus upon client acquisition.

For practices looking to extract additional funds from

their existing patients via Revenue Cycle Management (RCM), we ask to be compensated us as a base amount for total medical billing / coding (around 6.5% of billings) and a percentage of **increased** top-line revenue (25%). Practices only interested in acquiring new patients can opt to pay us a flat-monthly-fee between $3,000 and $7,500 plus whatever Google and Facebook ad spend will help the practice increase gross revenue.

Also, in some instances, we may ask for a 1-3% success fee up to a certain cap for any M&A transaction where we assist in advising the doctor who is acquiring or being acquired by another practice. If we provide funding for a practice acquisition, we may make a fee on that provision of capital.

(we will refer these fees to business brokers and banks if there is an evident conflict of interest or if the receipt of fees require licensure in certain states.)

If ever we are compensated in another manner, we will disclose this to our clients and allow them to opt-out if they wish.

We never disclose client contact information without permission and agree to a mutual non-disclosure clause with every client.

- **Do you guarantee that I will achieve the results that I want?**

Yes and no.

For our six-month lookback Revenue Cycle Management (RCM) audit, we will guarantee and increase in revenue or we will not charge the physician, period. Most of the money we make for this service is based upon INCREASED top-line revenue (see Chapter 1 for a hypothetical practice's example.)

For patient acquisition efforts, we do not guarantee results because there are so many parameters in play, from the talent of the doctor to the competitiveness of the geography, to the willingness for the doctor to reinvest in his or her practice (in the form of Google, Facebook and Instagram ads) as well as their general level of coachability.

Be wary of any guarantee that you are offered for Internet marketing. Total and complete certainty in Internet marketing-scenarios is often a sign of a lower intelligence on behalf of the Internet marketer, or someone who doesn't have the capacity to understand or discipline to assess all of the interdependent factors.

Due to the highly competitive nature of our clients' businesses, we've taken the time to document our processes and success for a single client and have posted that on our website as a case study. Our process is largely the same for new clients but may differ slightly depending upon in which practice they specialize.

So, those are real answers to the real questions. Be wary of answers that sound too idyllic and pay special attention to the detail of the answers. If it's a verbal conversation, the coach should be able to give a multitude of examples of HOW he or she accomplished what they claim to have accomplished.

Okay, here are now five questions that you should be prepared to answer in case your prospective coach asks to see if the fit would be a good one. I'll add answers to these questions that I would ultimately like to see from an ideal client candidate that you can model a bit if they apply to you (but please be truthful!):

- **What did you want to do before you realized that you wanted to become a doctor?**

    I wanted to play professional baseball. I played all through little league and high school. I really fell in love with the camaraderie that I experienced with my teammates and realized that nobody was better than anyone else. We all had our positions to play on the team and if any of us failed, we would all likely fail. So, we helped each other win.

- **What do you love most about being a doctor?**

    I enjoy seeing a client get better. I like to see them replace their troubled expression with a smile after they see what I am telling them is true and the healing or transformation has begun to take place. I love when they realize that there is a light at the end of the tunnel, and they are close to getting what they wanted when they first came in to see me.

- **What kind of billing / collections is your medical practice doing currently and what is your ultimate goal? What kind of net margin do you have after paying yourself?**

    We are currently billing approximately $105,000 per month and collecting around $65,000. We would like to be billing at least triple that with a collection's percentage over 90%. We are currently at about 12% net profit after I subtract my salary.

- **What makes your practice different than the practice down the street?**

We are really trying to figure that out right now. What I can tell you is that we have an amazing staff and they are fantastic at treating our customers like family. We do really great work but don't really know how best to leverage that to our best advantage to get more high-value patients.

- **Do you want to grow the practice organically, sell it outright or grow by buying out your competitors?**

Well, we'd really like to do all three. We'd like to grow organically and use some of that cash flow to leverage into buying a couple of practices in our geography, then once we are big enough, I'd like to sell the practices to a larger regional competitor or to a private equity fund.

See how the answers to those questions are direct and informative?

Both parties have a pretty darn good idea of what the other one wants and if and how they can help. All cards are on the table, no trickery or deception. Is it a good fit or not? Shall we do this or revisit another time?

## Final Word on Coaches

Now you have an idea of what to look for in a coach and what a coach may be looking for in you. Take your time to learn about your potential coaches, buy their book(s) and read them if they've taken the time and effort to write one. If they haven't written one in the topical area where you need help, ask yourself (and perhaps ask them) why they haven't written a book on the topic.

Finally, know that humans are fallible and that even superhuman coaches can make mistakes, your coach will make mistakes in advising you and you will make mistakes in executing the advice that your coach provides.

These mistakes will happen, so you must do what you can on a macro decision-making level to not make a major mistake when picking your coach.

In the words of the now-immortal *Trillionaire-Coach Bill Campbell: "Don't f*** it up."*

Mr. Nicholas Shawn Chavez

## PART II: BUILD

*Go placidly amid the noise and haste,*
*and remember what peace there may be in silence.*
*As far as possible without surrender*
*be on good terms with all persons.*
*Speak your truth quietly and clearly;*
*and listen to others,*
*even the dull and the ignorant;*
*they too have their story.*

*Avoid loud and aggressive persons,*
*they are vexations to the spirit.*
*If you compare yourself with others,*
*you may become vain and bitter;*
*for always there will be greater and lesser persons than yourself.*
*Enjoy your achievements as well as your plans.*

*Keep interested in your own career, however humble;*
*it is a real possession in the changing fortunes of time.*
*Exercise caution in your business affairs;*
*for the world is full of trickery.*
*But let this not blind you to what virtue there is;*
*many persons strive for high ideals;*
*and everywhere life is full of heroism...*

Derived from Max Ehrman's *Desiderata*, as recited to the author Nicholas Chavez at the age of 38 by his eldest son, Nicko Alexander who was then age 18.

## CHAPTER 7

# Principles of Digital Scale

I've always been a numbers guy, and my friends tell me I can actually tell a decent story from time to time. Usually those who can tell stories love to listen to stories, and I think that I am good with certain numbers because I can understand the stories that they try to tell me.

In fact, I know this to be true. I can recall almost any number or figure that I've heard that was uttered in the context of a subject that I cared about. I can almost always remember dollar figures associated with annual revenue, profit margins, COGS, EBITDA for nearly any business I've ever consulted for. Why? Because those numbers tell stories.

Contrast that with my inability to remember other numbers like someone's phone number, my PO BOX number, various zip codes for my credit card billing addresses or most other of what I consider to be non-contextual numbers. I really have to strain to remember people's names for the same reason, but I can almost always recall their profession or the city in which they live.

### A Ferrari or $200k Cash?

Sometimes, our brains do funny things with numbers. If someone were to ask you if you'd rather have a million dollars or a billion dollars, you'd probably pick the billion dollars because your brain knows that it's bigger. If I asked you if you wanted a brand new, shiny red Ferrari F8 Tributo or $200,000 in cash which would you pick? I'm guessing it would depend on your priorities and your knowledge of that particular Ferrari.

If you picked the cash, it's probably because you thought: "*Wow! I could pay off my student loans and a big chunk of my mortgage with that!*" Or, "*I sure would like to invest that $200k in cryptocurrency.*" The issue is, you'd have made the wrong choice because you made a choice based upon imperfect information.

Had you known that the model that the F8 Tributo replaced was the Ferrari 488 that had a base price of around $250,000 and that the F8 would likely sell substantially upward of MSRP for the next several years making its value (especially in the color that enthusiasts term "resale red") you'd have known that you were taking delivery of a car that could be sold within about a day or two for around $300,000 in cash, a 50% premium to simply accepting the $200,000 cash bundle.

Now imagine making this decision 1,000 times per day. To make 50% more money than you might otherwise have *at scale*, meaning that you can do it over and over and over again. Let's say that I charged you $10,000 every time you made a transaction. Now your profit drops from $100,000 to $90,000, but you can rely on the information to make 1,000 transactions per day. That's $90 million dollars per day.

That is the power of monetizing information and it's how the rich get rich and stay rich: it's called *arbitrage*.

Now it's a bit of a silly example because no single person or corporate entity could ever get an allocation of 1,000 Ferrari F8 Tributos, let alone in a single day; but, I've found that it's sometimes better to use a silly, easy to understand example than it is to lecture in an erudite, pedantic way about subject matter that might be factually correct but utterly boring and complex.

Okay, so you can't get 1,000 Ferraris a day and sell them. Let's think of another idea. What scales well? Ah. Digital products like software and music and movies. Stuff you can download right? Once you finish the product, it costs nearly the same to sell one as it does a million of them. But, unless you are the rare MD, DO, DDS, DMD or other doctor that knows how to code or shoot independent movies or rap like Eminem, that idea is out.

Hm. Wait. What else do you control?

Your time. Okay, this is not a great example because your time doesn't scale. You personally have 24 hours per day. Not more and not less; however, do you remember what we talked about in Chapter 6? Oprah scaled her time, right? How? Oprah hired 12,554 people to do her bidding every single day to command 301,296 hours of productivity per day to achieve a personal net worth of $2.5 billion.

Oh? You're not Oprah you say? Of course not. I'm not either. Only Oprah is Oprah, but that doesn't mean that you can't scale your business to get rich or even fantastically rich.

## A Billion Dollar Dentist

I recognized the house immediately as I browsed Instagram. I had always admired this home because I once lived in something that looked very similar to it from a design perspective. Only mine was about 29,000 square feet smaller and didn't include a backyard waterpark, or even a single basketball court (this house had two).

The owner had placed his and his wife's 35,000+ square foot estate up for sale a few years back for over $30 million and hunted for a buyer for years, without success, even after dropping the asking price by more than $8 million in that time to just a touch under $24 million. The house is probably the most majestic home I've ever seen and think it would easily qualify as a palace in other parts of the world, and perhaps it would qualify as such in the United States if it weren't crass to refer to one's home in such grandiose terms.

What did the homeowner do to earn this life of luxury? Let's break it down into some easy-to read bullets:

- A man started out as a dentist that founded a dental practice

- Based on the success of the single practice, the dentist went and found funding to build or buy more dental practices

- The dentist and his wife took the funding and their expertise and replicated the success they had at the single practice into several dozen regional locations

- The couple managed the practices as they opened over 50 locations under their umbrella

- After eight years, the couple sold 100% of the company to a private equity firm for a reported exit of more than a billion dollars.

Regardless of whether you agree with the way the couple accumulated their wealth or take umbrage with some of the methods that they'd reportedly used to generate billings for their dental centers, the you should focus on the following synopsis:

> With some excellent advice and help from his dedicated spouse, a dentist scaled-up a dental practice into over four-dozen locations and sold those practices for a nice multiple to a private equity shop.
>
> At some juncture after the sale, the former dentist was reported

*to be worth a billion dollars or thereabouts.*

If he did It as a doctor, you can do it as a doctor also. You just need to decide what you want, how much you want and whether you want to invest the time, energy and money necessary to win at that level.

You can do it. Make a plan, get some good advice and get it done.

## The $12.8 Billion Dollar Doctor

If one is the loneliest number, why not add another eleven-point-eight? With a 2019 fortune estimated at over $12.8 billion, Dr. Thomas Frist Jr. is the wealthiest doctor in the United States. Some of you may even have been employed by some of the 117 hospitals or 119 surgery centers under the HCA Healthcare umbrella that Dr. Frist founded with his father Dr. Thomas Frist, Sr. in 1968.

Okay, let's get the excuses out of the way now: *"Well Nicholas, 1968 was a long time ago. It was a simpler time in medicine."* or, *"Well, he had the help of his dad and I am flying solo without a family fortune at my back."*

Those are both excuses. Lame excuses at that.

Let me rebut them one at a time for your benefit; first, yes 1968 was a half-century ago and I'll agree that medicine was certainly simpler then, but so were the capital markets.

## 1968 Was Long Ago?

Let's get the statistics out of the way: there were roughly a third as many doctors in the United States in 1968 than there are now, and since that time the United States population has grown by nearly half. Then the ratio of doctors to potential patients in the United States was approximately 1 physician per

Mr. Nicholas Shawn Chavez

623 U.S. citizens, now there is approximately 1 physician per 328 U.S. citizens. Despite the favorable increase in the number of doctors to care for patients, I think we would be hard-pressed to find anyone who thinks patients are better served as a 2019 aggregate than their 1968 counterparts were (controlling for advancements in medical technology of course).

I understand. Being a general practitioner paid better back then; but options exist today for the doctor-entrepreneur that did not exist back in the 60's. The primary enabling factor for these opportunities is capital in the form of private equity and venture capital.

In 1968, private equity was in its infancy and the time was right to prepare for an initial public offering of stock for HCA when it had a comparatively small inventory of medical facilities numbering less than a dozen in total.

Note that my former client, private equity giant Kohlberg Kravis Roberts (KKR) would not be founded for a decade AFTER this transaction. KKR would eventually assist in the syndication of a "go-private" acquisition (alongside fellow PE titan Bain Capital and Merrill Lynch) of HCA Healthcare of more than $33.6 billion.

While I cannot speak for them, I know beyond a shadow of a doubt that KKR looks for synergistic acquisitions on a daily basis in the medical field and they have the process down to a science now. They are looking to make returns for their limited partners and shareholders, and in the process, they will make a handful of doctors incredibly wealthy. Perhaps some of those doctors will become billionaires and as instrumental in American politics as the Frist family has become.

There has never been more liquidity in the American economy than there is now as we begin the third decade of the 21$^{st}$ century. This liquidity is tirelessly hunting for stable investments that will produce higher-than-average yield. Health Care fits this model very well, so even though you might long for a simpler time in medicine as a practitioner, you could not be more advantageously positioned in the history of time as a capitalist.

## No Help?

I've written the outline for a book that has been knocking around my brain for a while that is an examination of people who have obtained success by the standard of American society, and what, if any help they had from their family to get there.

For now, in absence of the book being written, let's agree that it does seem to be of inordinate help to have a close family member who is skilled and already successful in any industry one wishes to conquer. The alignment of familial self-interest is seemingly due to deep-rooted evolutionary psychology of resource attainment. This multi-generational effort to secure a top ranking in competitive genetics is certainly a tough combination of factors to beat.

But, it's not unbeatable.

You have to make up your mind to subjugate your own ego and share the pie. You need to look for an intelligent, enthusiastic business partner who understands health care economics, the intricate details that surround relevant aspects of capital markets and fast-evolving technology. The combination of your skill as a passionate doctor and the skill of an unstoppable economist could be far more powerful than that of a generationally structured family partnership.

Why?

Simple. Urgency.

People like us realize that there is no time to waste and that anything that we have in this world we must reach out and grasp for ourselves.

There is no waiting trust fund, we'll not be handed the keys to a publicly-traded entity or a hospital that was erected by our forebears. We must simply wake earlier, grind harder, partner smarter while out executing the blue bloods who seek to keep the best for themselves[11].

You've probably heard that "old-money" families have a certain distaste for families that are newly moneyed. Old money will claim the new money is brash, unrefined and non-sophisticated; the reality is that the entrance of a new family into the moneyed circle represents a (perhaps unwelcomed) change in what once was.

Take the time to find enthusiastic, smart & educated partners. It can pay literal dividends.

## Beating the Odds

Just with these two billionaire examples out of the aggregate population of approximately 200,000 dentists and 1.1 million physicians recorded as active in the United in 2018, the odds are roughly 1 in ~650,000 that a dentist or a doctor the U.S. can become a billionaire by scaling his or her practice using intelligent operational efficiencies and private equity.

Those are not long odds, especially when compared with the odds of winning Powerball at 1 in ~292 million.

The most evident differentiator is that, to my knowledge, no one can tell you how to win the Powerball; however, there are multiple examples of doctors who have scaled their medical and dental practices to achieve lottery-sized payouts.

To take action, a doctor must decide that this type of wealth is what he or she wants. The next action is to build his or her team to begin to scale, but take caution: *there are snakes in the grass.*

## CHAPTER 8

## On Internet Marketers

Man. This is a tough chapter to write.

In Chapter 6 we talked about the dubious business model of a certain doctor who was compensated for referring an Internet marketer to his client-doctors who trusted him as a "coach" and we walked through probable compensation. In the next section, we will talk a little about a few fictional Internet marketing companies that may have some striking similarities to some that are out there in the real world, including the one that the doctor "coach" was referring for allegedly undisclosed referral fees.

I am writing this chapter as a guide for you to delineate the good Internet marketers from the bad. Primarily because I predict Internet marketing *really is the engine that drives new patient acquisition in the 2020's & 2030's* and also partially because Internet marketing as an industry has been sullied by hucksters.

**Put simply, most Internet marketers suck.** They are bad people with bad intentions: they are grifters who want a lot of money to deliver little value. They target doctors, wrongly thinking that they are "rich."

So, I'm going to tell you how to identify good ones and stay away from the bad ones.

Factually, I have put off writing this chapter for two weeks, literally looking for any other possible "priority" to address in its place. I suspect that I am feeling significant reticence here because I am going to put forth some unpopular facts that will win me little affection from some who would call themselves competitors to DigitalGoals (I would not classify them as such.)

While I will not name names, I will tell true stories while obscuring certain identifying detail to reduce the possibility of being sued by the offending parties. Due to the evidence I possess, I no doubt would win any lawsuit, but it would be a pyrrhic victory at best given the expected time and effort involved.

You'll just have to use your imagination while piecing together the detail that is intentionally left out of some of these stories.

Fortunately for me the truth is an absolute defense against allegations of defamation and if any of these stories were true, you could bet your bottom dollar I could (and would) prove their veracity, or I wouldn't have taken the risk to write them down.

## Here's Jonny!

*Here's a hypothetical based upon real people and events with names, locations, specialties and details changed:*

Let's talk about a fictional Internet marketer named Jon Michaels from New Hampshire. Jon is a pleasantly plump extrovert with a persistent grin and a hearty handshake. He likes cigars, sports cars, boats and golf. When he flies, he often charters a jet (though at those astronomical prices only God knows why.)

When you meet him, you instantly like him. His smile and cherubic face are disarming, he's soft spoken without being meek. You believe him when he tells you that he's been building websites since high school, and he smiles warmly when he asks you to call him "Jonny" since "none of his real friends call him Jon."

Jonny was introduced to you by another doctor from Chicago named Justin, that you know like and trust. In fact, you've been paying Dr. Justin to coach you on the finer points of your practice since you share a specialty with him in rheumatology he seems to know what he's talking about since he's written a handful of books and lectured at a local college in certain topics that pertain to your mutual practices.

Jonny offers you a "trial deal" of a few months of his Internet marketing service but insists that you need a website redesign that costs somewhere between $15,000 and $30,000. His fee is several thousand a month and he urges you to spend another few thousand on pay-per-click (PPC) ads with Google and Facebook. He brags about his high client retention percentage (to a very specific percentage, which never seems to change) but doesn't give any data to back it up, you don't ask for it because you don't want to seem rude and you really want Jonny's new Internet marketing system to work well for you. (Plus, he's SO cool!)

Despite the fact that you think your website is already pretty darn good, you acquiesce and allow Jonny's team to rebuild your website, a task that takes around three months.

Let's dive in a little deeper.

## Lambo Livin!

It would be in somewhat poor taste for Jonny to take selfies and blast them all over the Internet with his big house, private jets and brand-new exotic cars before he ensured that his clients were protected from basic but important policy infractions (like HIPAA) right?

Yes. One would think.

I remember seeing my first REAL exotic car (on television) in 1999 when I was just out of high school. A then-unknown, 28-

year-old Elon Musk purchased a McLaren F1 for around a million dollars after selling his company to the entity that would eventually become PayPal.

This was a significant trophy, and one that Elon sacrificed for.

Opting to use the majority of his liquidity to purchase it "instead of a house in Palo Alto" where he ended up buying a modestly priced condo instead. Nearly two decades later a McLaren of that model and vintage is worth in excess of $15 million and Elon is a billionaire.

Jonny drives a Lamborghini, though in comparison to Elon's McLaren, it is a mass-produced model. Another sharp comparison is that Jonny didn't pay cash for his after a successful exit of his company, he financed it with 20% down and pays around $2,500 per month for the privilege of driving it in addition to another exotic car that he owned simultaneously for a time, a convertible Maserati Granturismo. The Maserati was financed in a similar manner.

Now, I am happy that we live in the U.S. and that we can spend our money as we please. I've admitted to previously owning and enjoying a Ferrari F355 GTS that I later sold in 2007 to the Ferrari dealer after experiencing some of the now infamous issues with its headers and valve guides.

So, why do I bring up Johnny's Lambo? Do I hate capitalism?

Nah. I'm just pointing out his margins and utter disregard for his client-doctors' business by endangering them with HIPAA violations, instead choosing to focus on rewarding himself lavishly while his clients are at risk.

*Capitalism doesn't hurt people. Ego and ignorance hurts people.*

We all know that the basics of business work by buying something, for a dollar and then selling it for two. If you pay a dental associate or a nurse practitioner as part of your dental or medical practice, you are doing it also. Yay capitalism! Good stuff!

However, we've all heard of stories where people are hurt through the sale of substandard materials that end up hurting end-consumers, right? Lately, the culprits have been cosmetics, toys and dogfood sourced from China. These products were discovered to hold high quantities of lead and were literally killing children and their pets with lead or other toxic chemical poisoning. Why would anyone paint a toy with lead paint? Why would anyone allow lead to infiltrate cosmetics applied to one's lips or the food source for an animal?

The reason is ego. More specifically, the reason is *profit margin* to buy more stuff to feed an ego.

Lead is a cheap filler, and by utilizing lead as a material in place of a more expensive, less dangerous material, the manufacturer pays less, charges market price and keeps more of the money made from the sale.

I can hear you ask: *"Okay, so what does Jonny's Lambo have to do with the price of lead in China?"*

Very simply, Jonny is using substandard material or subcontractor services to fulfill his commitment to his clients; specifically, in the manner of web hosting and advertising services. The reason this is important is because the hosting that Jonny is using has not been certified as HIPAA compliant, and the Facebook advertising method that Jonny's subcontractors are using has violated HIPAA in a major way by uploading actual patient data to Facebook for monetary gain.

## HIPAA Compliant Hosting Violations

We offer two types of HIPAA compliant hosting for our Elite 300 clients. One is for their website, and the other is for their artificial-intelligence enabled call-tracking software that enables data mining to figure out, say, all the patients that called in about a dental implant or a rhinoplasty that month.

It's scary cool stuff, and because of the sensitivity of that data, we spend a significant amount of money to ensure that data is housed on a HIPAA compliant server on behalf of our clients and their patients.

What if this data wasn't housed on a HIPAA compliant server?

What if the server was shared and your competitors laid their hands on the information?

What if it were a hacker that stole and sold your patients private health information data on a black-market website on the dark web?

Worse, what if a nation-state hacker was aggregating patient data for targets who held a certain ailment for an eventual coordinated exposure to a disability or death inducing agent?

These sound like pretty far out concerns, but I can assure you that I've spent enough time in conversation with certain government agencies to know that these scenarios are not only possible, but that they are probable in the long run.

A great way to know if your Internet marketer is hosting your site or call tracking system on a HIPAA compliant server is whether they sent you a HIPAA Business Associate Agreement (BAA) to sign. You may also ask to see the BAA that they signed with the ultimate cloud / hosting provider.

Do you think that Jonny had his clients sign a BAA from him when they were sold? I sure hope so. You can't be too careful here.

## Potential Jail-time for Facebook Violations

HIPAA hosting is important, and not having your website and call tracking hosted on a HIPAA compliant server does not always put your practice out of compliance, and I am pretty sure that you wouldn't have government agents breaking down your door if word of the violation got out. If patient data was somehow exposed in a breach, you'd probably get hit with a nominal fine and given a short amount of time to get your act together with your Internet hosting provider since HIPAA compliance ultimately falls upon the doctor first.

The Facebook violations we will talk about here are grave. They are intentionally-made errors that are both simultaneously difficult to detect and carry a possibility of both bankrupting and incarcerating a doctor.

*Take this hypothetical into account:*

A plastic surgeon hires Jonny to do Internet marketing for the purpose of bringing in more rhinoplasty patients in the Beverly Hills area. Jonny says he can accomplish this through Facebook advertising, but the clicks or "conversions" will be expensive due to the high level of competition for plastic surgeons in the Beverly Hills geographic area. Leads coming in through Facebook to the doctor's webpage or "landing" page will cost anywhere between $100 and $300 per click!

Jonny knows that his new client doesn't want to waste money on Facebook clicks from existing rhinoplasty patients, so he asks the plastic surgeon for an existing patient list. The surgeon provides the list, happy to exclude current patients who might cost him up to $300 per click without generating a new patient relationship.

Jonny provides this list to his subcontractor who may or may not be overseas. This subcontractor is not a specialist in plastic surgery and is not aware of medical regulation or policy in the United States since this subcontractor may fulfill Facebook ads for a great number of clients in varied industries such as country clubs, jewelry stores and car dealerships.

At Jonny's request the subcontractor uploads the patient list to Facebook to create both a "Facebook Custom Audience" and a "Exclusion List". The Custom Audience allows the Facebook algorithm to find persons similar to the patient lists, comparing income, household size, profession and other demographics. The Exclusion List simply enables Facebook to hide the ad from the existing patient base to ensure there isn't a negative return on investment (ROI) from existing patients clicking the ad and not converting into new revenue.

*"What's the big deal about that?"* you ask. *"Who cares if Facebook has the name or email address of my patient?"*

Dang! It's a big deal!

Here's why: Facebook aggregates a LOT of data about every single user, who they know, where they live, where they go, what they talk about, what their sentiment is about certain topics, what brands they like, what television shows they watch, which celebrities that they adore, etc.

Imagine Facebook knowing that a user has had a medical procedure. This is data that other marketers would pay a LOT of money for to sell them other items. While this potential barrage of ancillary ads may be irritating, it is not the core issue.

The core issue is doctor-patient confidentiality. What if we weren't talking about rhinoplasty and instead were talking about a plastic surgeon who specialized in penile enlargement?

Mr. Nicholas Shawn Chavez

How would those patients feel if they knew that their identifying information had been uploaded to Facebook?

What if we weren't talking about a plastic surgeon at all, and instead we were discussing a sexually transmitted disease (STD) clinic that was hoping to drum up new business?

It's a problem. The framers and implementers of HIPAA seemed to know that data would be commercially valuable, and as such assigned a MASSIVE fiscal and criminal penalty to violations that may fit this particular mold:

> *42 U.S. Code §1320d–6. Wrongful disclosure of individually identifiable health information*
>
> *(a) Offense*
>
> *A person who knowingly and in violation of this part—*
>
> *(1) uses or causes to be used a unique health identifier;*
>
> *(2) obtains individually identifiable health information relating to an individual; or*
>
> *(3) discloses individually identifiable health information to another person, shall be punished as provided in subsection*
>
> *(b). For purposes of the previous sentence, a person (including an employee or other individual) shall be considered to have obtained or disclosed individually identifiable health information in violation of this part if the information is maintained by a covered entity (as defined in the HIPAA privacy regulation described in section 1320d–9(b)(3) of this title) and the individual obtained or disclosed such information without authorization.*
>
> *(b) Penalties*

*A person described in subsection (a) shall—*

*(1) be fined not more than $50,000, imprisoned not more than 1 year, or both;*

*(2) if the offense is committed under false pretenses, be fined not more than $100,000, imprisoned not more than 5 years, or both; and*

*(3) if the offense is committed with intent to sell, transfer, or use individually identifiable health information for commercial advantage, personal gain, or malicious harm, be fined not more than $250,000, imprisoned not more than 10 years, or both.*

The real question is whether or not the U.S. Attorney for whatever district where the doctor practiced interpreted saving up-to-$300 per existing-patient who was excluded from clicking an ad on Facebook was a "commercial advantage" or a "personal gain."

If Jonny discussed the reasoning behind this with the doctor prior to getting the patient list, or the execution parameters with the subcontractor (if U.S. based) then the doctor may very well be on the hook for the criminal penalties.

I'll ask again: *"Do you have a BAA signed with your Internet marketing provider?"*

If you don't, why don't you? Are you aware of anything that might have been done with your patient list or patient files? *I'd heartily recommend giving us a call if you cannot remember signing a BAA with your Internet marketer. We can help protect you.*

If you think this chapter is just a trumped-up scare tactic, spend a few minutes Googling around to understand the extent of the doctors and dentists who have been fined and jailed for these types of violations.

Even if neither of those penalties were on the table, is risking your reputation worth it? I'd imagine not. You worked hard to get where you are.

If you approach your Internet marketer with this information and they stall, or don't produce what you are looking for- call us immediately and we will sign a BAA that very day with you and begin the migration of your web presence and call tracking to our HIPAA compliant servers. *To ease the transition, if your practice qualifies, we will beat your current Internet marketer's monthly fee structure by at least 8% while ensuring that you are compliant.*

If any investigation or lawsuit happens at a later time, you can point to the BAA that you signed with DigitalGoals as the "immediate corrective action" that you took when you learned that there might be HIPAA violations being incurred by your Internet marketer. This will be important if a civil or criminal case is filed to keep your reputation pristine and stay far afield of accusations of wrongdoing.

Our 8% discount will add up favorably for you, and 90% of the time we do not need to rebuild your website. We often waive startup fees for practices transferring from a non-HIPAA compliant Internet marketer as a courtesy, since they've likely been burned pretty badly and are already worried about the integrity of their practice.

Finally, the lesser, but still satisfying benefit is that your current Internet marketer will no longer get to laugh all the way to the bank in his shiny Lamborghini.

## CHAPTER 9

## Real Patient Acquisition

I am so thrilled to be writing this chapter.

Not only so we can jointly shake of the negativity of Chapter 8, but because *this is where we shine*.

This is where we make money ethically, legally and in compliance with federal regulations. ***This is where we win together!***

What we do is incredibly difficult work. It takes hard work, intelligence, insight and persistence. For that reason, I'm nearly willing to lay our process bare to allow anyone who wishes to try to replicate it to make an attempt to do so. My bet is that they would fail. The work is just too detailed and difficult for a weekend warrior to hope to eclipse our results, it is quite literally hundreds of steps long and requires the coordinated effort of many dozens of talented people.

But, I am not going to go through hundreds of steps here for two reasons:

1. Our clients pay for exclusivity, it is not in their best interests to put forth 100% of the knowledge necessary to achieve the results that they pay a significant sum for.

2. I imagine that as a doctor or dentist, you are quite busy with your patient base and you are looking for a general education to enable you to make intelligent decisions about matters relating to growing your practice through the intelligent hiring of vendors and partners.

As such, I will describe key steps in our process with a level of detail that should ensure a thorough understanding, but not so thorough to expose some of the secrets that our future Elite 300 clients will come to rely on daily for outsized returns.

## Your Web Presence

When most Internet marketers talk about your "web presence" they are referring to your "website." Rookie and low-level marketers use these terms interchangeably, relying their targets' unfamiliarity with the topic of Internet marketing to overcharge them for a website. In truth, a website is central to your web presence, but contrary to what these Internet marketers pitch you, it might not be the most important aspect of your web presence.

Now I'm going to hit you with some truth: **_YOU PROBABLY DO NOT NEED A NEW "CUSTOM" WEBSITE._**

You might *want* a new custom website which is a different matter entirely. We can talk about why you might want a new website a bit later in this section; but first let's explore the reasoning regarding not "needing" a new website.

Regretfully, most marketers will try to sell you a brand-new website as part of their "marketing package." Some spikey-haired-Internet-marketers go so far as to say that they "will not help" companies who do not commit to a full website redesign. This is poor guidance and as you might imagine, is designed to extract dollars from clients in a major way. Even if your current website is perfectly acceptable and just needs a bit of a tune up, *they will advocate for rebuilding the ENTIRE site.* This would be like popping a brand-new engine in your car when all you needed was a few of the critical parts replaced with improved versions. It's wasteful and time consuming.

# RICH DOCS

*I'm not too proud to admit that we learned this lesson the hard way.*

For our first Elite 300 client, we did a full website redesign. We re-did everything from the text content to the photos, to the 3D images. We built 21 new videos and custom moving image content for the headers. We sourced a new domain and new SSL certificate for secure transactions. We had a HIPAA compliant server built.

It was quite naturally excellent from a technical perspective with all of the proper meta data for the Google search engine spiders to crawl for all of the pages, as well as the images and videos.

Now, we didn't try to "upsell" this client on a new site in order to get a bigger payout from their deal. As a matter of fact, we did so much work that we were largely upside-down on the deal from a financial perspective in the beginning because we wanted everything to be *perfect.*

Our team was devastated when the practice told us they weren't satisfied with the site. They said that the "look and feel" wasn't quite what they had agonized over and finally settled upon with their former site and that they felt that the verbiage promised patient results a bit too aggressively for their comfort.

We offered them three go-forward options:

1. We would make their changes to the redesigned site. This process would surely have taken a great deal of time; possibly a month or more due to the reliance on the client to give development feedback and iterate. Selecting this option would likely yield the best results from a technical search engine optimization perspective.

2. We could apply everything about the "new" site that they liked to their "old" site. This wouldn't be quick but would preserve their brand ethos while taking advantage of much of the new technology and content that we created. From a technical search engine optimization perspective, this would not offer the best result, but would provide for a notable improvement in their existing Google ranking.

3. We could transfer all the code and content that we developed to another firm of their choosing that could implement it selectively on their behalf, we would also waive certain fees owed and provide them a refund of unused PPC spend. We could clearly not foresee the technical search engine optimization results here because we would have no idea which provider they might choose.

The client chose, in their words "door number two."

Let's examine why the second option was selected. It seems that the Operations Manager for the five-location practice took "hundreds of hours" to build their existing website, making sure to focus on the detailed "look and feel" that they wanted to present as a practice.

To be fair, their old website was warm and friendly and was a natural extension of the welcoming feel that they strove to envelop their patients in when they walked through the doors of the practice.

The primary issue was that their old website, especially the home page, did not pass the *Brand X Test*.

## The Brand X Test

You remember *Brand X* from all the prime-time television commercials, right? Laundry detergent, soft-drinks, trash bags, diapers all pitted brand name items against items from Brand X.

Usually, by the end of the 30 or 60 second commercial, viewers would never go with the generic Brand X version, preferring to go with the capability and quality of the name brand.

*The Brand X Test* is where you load up your site and cover up your practice's logo and ask yourself, "could this be any other practice in the world?" For most sites, including our client's, the answer was yes.

Site visitors were immediately greeted with the image of a smiling family with perfect white smiles, playing in a green park on a sunny day. Platitudes about how the practice "cared for its patients" were featured prominently near the images. As I'd said, the site was warm and friendly; it was certainly geared to human-readership for those who already knew about the practice, but it had a few critical flaws from a patient-prospect perspective.

The primary issue was that the home page of the original client site could have been a website for *any-other-dental-practice-on Earth.* Unfortunately, it could also have been a website for a medical practice, a health insurance company, a college-savings plan, or an adoption agency.

When patient-prospects visit a site, they want to immediately experience *congruence* meaning that the pictures and the words that are on the home page should match the pictures and the words that they have in their brain when they are searching for a solution to a problem.

Are they looking for braces for their teen? They should see braces when they click on your site. Are they hoping to have a face-lift? They should see photos of smiling post-op patients or a motion image showing a patient having a happy and productive consultation with the surgeon.

## Sell Disney World?

Have you ever heard a marketer admonish something to the effect of "Sell Disney World, not the flight to Orlando"?

I get it. Families who travel to Florida to experience the *House of the Mouse* do not care a whole lot about how they get there, they are thinking about the end results of making memories with their family and taking photos that they will look at after brunch in 20-30 years with their grandchildren.

But they still need to get to Orlando.

What most marketers do not understand is that you must alleviate the worried thoughts of the buyer before the buyer can really sell him or herself on the pleasure that they will receive from the experience. An intelligent travel agent will of course show pictures of a family happily strolling from attraction-to-attraction inside a flowered, sunny Disney World; but they will also address the logistical details in a near-immediate manner.

For example, if a travel agent is selling a "Disney World All Inclusive Package" the best photos to use on their website, is a photo of a happy family on a plane, in a rental car, checking into a hotel AND FINALLY a family happily strolling from attraction-to-attraction inside a flowered, sunny Disney World.

You need to tell the complete story. You must make it easy for your prospective patient to get from Point A in their mind: "I want to get this procedure done to feel better about myself" to Point B: "Wow, it seems like it's pretty easy to get this procedure done… I guess it's worth a phone call…"

Sell Disney World, and the flight, and the hotel and the rental car.

Sell the package!

This will look different for every practice, whether it be medical or dental, but let's take an example we can all follow since most of us have kids we care for and because we love them we are eager to spend money to make sure they have a beautiful smile. Beautiful smiles usually mean one thing: braces.

Do we have to show a teenage kid with a seriously crooked smile as a starting point to the story? Nah. Just like the Disney World travel agent wouldn't need to show you frustrated with your job and in need of a vacation. You already know that you need a break, just like you already know that your kid's teeth are something that might get him made-fun-of if you don't get it fixed before he graduates high school.

We can start in the ortho's office. Maybe the mom or dad (or both) is sitting there listening intently to the orthodontist talk about options, we see Junior sitting in the chair with a closed-lipped smile. The next few photos are of the procedure being conducted and the final few pictures are of Junior out in the wild, showing his braces off confidently. If we are really feeling ambitious, we can show a photo after the braces have been removed, or better yet, a testimonial video featuring Junior and his loving parents gushing about how handsome their son's smile is.

That tells a better story to a prospective patient than a static photo of a family sitting in a green park on a sunny afternoon, right?

**Semi-Custom Home(pages)**

An ex of mine was fond of calling my former home a "McMansion" because in her mind, it wasn't a "true" mansion. I attributed this silly comment to a temporary mean spiritedness on her behalf.

Anyway, I never really figured out what she meant by this, considering it was a 6,500 square foot English Tudor that was built in the 1930s[12]. Perhaps she was referring to a "real" mansion as being something equivalent to the famed "Biltmore" mansion built in 1895 at a total square footage of 175,000 square feet. Either way, now that house is gone and so is she.

I now live in a smaller, more manageable semi-custom home. It's probably not even big enough to apply the puzzling McMansion label to, but wow is it ever easier to deal with!

My wife and I made a conscious decision to go semi-custom in a gated community because we could simply lock the door and leave it unattended for months at a time while we spend time in Manhattan, Colorado or elsewhere. We found that when we had a monstrous, expensive home we felt guilty not spending time there, because it felt wasteful to spend significant amounts of money to travel extensively while we were putting out substantial dollars for our primary residence to sit empty.

We don't miss most of the luxuries that we had there. We dropped down a few bedrooms, several fireplaces, several bathrooms (with urinals!) two bars and an extra oven; we also traded our golf-course view for a water view. All in, our current home is functionally nearly the same and cost about 20% of the Italianesque Travertine Monstrosity and the English Tudor before it and the French Provincial before it. The only thing I miss is the steam shower.

Why do I mention custom homes? Custom homes are like custom websites. They are cool, and they can be worthy of some serious bragging rights, but at the end of the day, they really don't function differently than a nicely-constructed semi-custom website that costs less and leaves money left over for other priorities such as medical and dental conferences, advertising or additional staff.

Let's examine the custom components needed to turn a template-track-home website equivalent into a semi-custom-home-on-a-lake-website without the need to spend custom-ocean-front-estate-website dollars.

Critical Components of a Successful Website:

1. Custom video interviews with every doctor in your practice
2. Procedure specific photos
3. Procedure specific written content
4. Dynamic phone numbers to track individual prospects
5. Site analytics to track visitor behavior
6. HIPAA compliant hosting

It should go without saying that all these aspects of your site should have the proper technical integrations to enable Google to process, sort and rank your content in an efficient and consistent manner. If you do not focus on this step, all the rest are for naught.

Now ask yourself this question: "Do I really need a new custom website at a cost of $20-30k or am I willing to spend $10-15k to get all of the custom media components necessary to turn my existing, template based website into a semi-custom website that brings in clients?"

Remember that every dollar that you save in the construction of your website is a dollar that can be put toward paid ads on Google or Facebook.

Don't skimp, but don't overpay. Your site is for getting new patients for your practice, don't let a pointy haired Internet marketer sell you more than you need, and don't let your ego overpay for a Biltmore size estate on the Internet when all you really need is a semi-custom 5 bedroom on the water.

## Citations: GMBs, NAPs and MAPs

Okay, citations are essentially collections of information about companies on the Internet. For those of you (like me) who are old enough to remember the Yellow Pages books, you can consider these NAPs as the new standard listings in the Yellow Pages, not the display ads mind you, just the name of the business, address and phone number.

These citations are referred to as by Internet marketers by one of a couple acronyms:

- NAP: Name Address and Phone Number

    This is a generic acronym for web citations and you can see that it includes the same information that would have been included in a telephone directory for free 20 years ago; however, these NAP citations are not "automatic" you actually have to set them up.

    They are a critical factor that influences which web directories show for people searching for that TYPE of business. So, if a competing practice in your town has their NAP setup and you don't, guess who Google or Bing or Yelp is going to send your customer to?

    That's right. You don't get the business... Dr. Smith across town who had someone setup his NAP does. Sad.

- GMB: Google My Business

    This is a Google-specific NAP listing, it's the one you see on the right-hand side of the search results page after you enter a company name into the Google Search Bar. It usually has the following information:

- Company Name
- Phone Number
- Physical Address
- Web Address
- Operating Hours
- Customer Ratings
- Reviews
- Location Photos
- Location Map / Driving Directions
- CID

There are a great many sites where a doctor should have his or her information input in standard NAP format, and all of these citations should be consistent for obvious reasons, not the least of which is that Google will check these citations for consistency and either increase or decrease your ranking based upon an accuracy score. Did you move locations for your practice? Update your citations. Did you change operating hours? Update your citations. Using a new call-tracking number? Update your citations.

Ignore this advice at the peril of your practice's top line revenue. The price of getting this wrong grows every day, as does the benefit of getting it right.

This topic is most readily and easily understood through an interactive demonstration. This is only fun if we all play together now so I'll ask your participation here. Ready?

1. Grab your phone
2. Open your maps app (the ones you get directions while traveling to and fro)
3. Enter in your business name

4. Hopefully you've received a match for your business in your hometown
5. Click "Get Directions"
6. If you have gotten directions to your practice from your current location, that means that you have at least one major NAP citation setup properly which is great, but you need to make sure that your citations are consistent and ubiquitous.

## 5 Star Ratings

I usually go to the same dozen or so restaurants and order a particular entrée at each of them that I know I will enjoy. I don't hunt around the menu for something new to try, I eat the same thing prepared the same way every single time, if I want something else, I will go to another restaurant and order the dish I like at that restaurant.

This is a sufficient amount of variety for me and it practically guarantees that I never eat a bad meal (you can see evidence of this around my midsection. I'm working on it. Promise.)

This systematic, limited selection of dining establishments is a constant source of mild aggravation for my lovely, adventurous wife Jes, who easily tires of the same fare. Her perfect evening would be to find a new restaurant that doesn't have a menu and empower the chef to prepare something that he or she is known for, without any input as to whether we would enjoy it or whether we might be allergic to the ingredients.

Thankfully, there is a grand adjudicator of our going-out-to-eat decisions and it is Google. Jes will Google the type of food that she is craving, and she knows that as long it has a rating of more than 4 stars and at least 30+ total reviews, I will agree (albeit reluctantly) to *try* the restaurant. If I like it and the dish I try, I will add it to my rotation of restaurant "regulars."

Admit it, you do something similar; but it might be when searching for an auto mechanic, a florist or a liquor store that hopefully carries the sometimes-difficult-to-find-pinot-noir that you like. You search for "_____ near me" or "_____ in" whatever city you happen to be in at the time.

You're a human. Your patients and prospective patients are humans also. They have smartphones and laptops, and they search for your business in the same way you search for their businesses. It's not magic. It's not different. It's the same. We all look for the same thing. **_We all look for as many 5-star ratings as possible._**

Why do we do this? We do it because it's a mental shortcut. After a long day at the office, we start in on our second wave of responsibilities: What to eat, where to live, what to buy, what dentist we will use, who our primary care physician will be, what kind of bike to buy, which car to lease, which book to read on which vacation we will take whenever we get our tax refund back from whichever CPA we choose to prepare our taxes.

You might be the doctor or dentist in this scenario. Do you meet my criteria of 30 reviews with a minimum four-star rating? It's an arbitrary number and everyone has their own litmus, and it might be different for a taco restaurant than it is for a place to get Botox injections.

For this reason, we implement either an automated third-party review and follow-up system for our clients or one directly from DigitalGoals (depending upon the type of practice) to generate as many 5-star-reviews as possible. A great aspect of the functionality is that the software will detect a negative review and email any review below the four-star threshold directly to your office manager or operations director to remediate quickly before the client posts the negativity directly to Google or another public-facing review site.

We then go through these reviews as part of the monthly strategy review with each of our Elite 300 clients. These reviews are important to increasing the top-line-revenue of our clients' practices, and eventually the exit multiple of the practice valuation upon sale.

## A Video is Worth 1.8 Million Words

Forrester Research is one of the biggest names in technical research alongside Gartner. Forrester's Dr. James McQuivey predicted the explosion of video on the Internet in 2008 and explained "if a video is worth 1,000 words, a video is worth 1.8 million." I'm not going to break down McQuivey's math here, so let's just agree that the new consumer spends a ton of time watching YouTube videos in order to educate and entertain themselves.

I am no mechanic, but after watching YouTube videos, I was able to find what ailed my rapidly-approaching-classic-age Jaguar XJR (a squeaking supercharger belt). How did I do this you might ask? Well, as useful as threaded discussions on forums and technical bulletins might be, they don't have any sound... and I needed to understand if my *squeak-squeak-squeak* sounded like anyone else's *squeak-squeak-squeak* and instead wasn't being mistaken for a *squeal-squeal-squeal*. A picture wouldn't have helped that diagnosis and an audio recording could have helped match the sound, but I wouldn't have seen a finger pointed toward the supercharger pulley. I also wouldn't have seen the helpful Englishman smile and say, "looks like the problem is right 'ere, up underneath the bonnet." So, maybe not 1.8 million words, but definitely more than 1,000 words.

Now, what if this video would have been on my local, independent Jaguar mechanic's website? I instantly would have known that she knew how to remedy the issue. This would have given me the confidence to know two things:

1. The specialist is aware of this particular issue with this particular car
2. She can probably fix it more efficiently than the Jaguar dealership

That's an easy sale. As I said, I'm not a mechanic. So even if the video would have listed in explicit detail the exact manner of replacing the supercharger belt, there is simply no-freaking-way I would attempt the repair, no matter how "easy" the English chappie on the video says it would be to accomplish. I'll take it to my indie Jag mechanic and pay him to fix it.

Video seals the deal for buying-intent on the Internet. This is why we make an extra effort to record our doctors' actual patients giving REAL testimonials about SPECIFIC procedures that they'd had done. They mention the doctors by name, they talk about the care they received by the staff at the practice, they glow about the results and always say that the procedure was "worth the money."

Done. That's going to sell half of the clients that you are the right doctor to complete the procedure, the rest is a matter of minor logistics and payment terms.

Google loves video too, for a few reasons:

- When users navigate to your website via a Google search, the Google search algorithm measures their "dwell time" or the amount of time they spend on your site before they click away to another site. The opposite measure of "dwell time" is "bounce rate" as in, if someone searches for "Chicago Cosmetic Surgeon" and they land on your site, don't see anything that captivates their interest and they "bounce" off of your site and onto another.

    Videos increase engagement and dwell time while correspondingly decreasing bounce rate.

- Google owns YouTube, so the Google search algorithm will often display YouTube videos as search results for queries typed into the Google search engine. Metrics matter to Google also, so they want to show their advertisers that they control as much of a user's interaction with the Internet as possible. This is why we currently host all of our client videos with YouTube as opposed to competitors Amazon, Vimeo or Wistia.

- Google videos embedded in the Google My Business (GMB) citation will increase the search engine rank result of that business because there is a lower probability that the business is a scam.

For all of these reasons (and a few more that we won't disclose here), we often use Emmy-award winning videographers to capture the very best angles, lighting and special moments from our Elite 300 clients and their patients to ensure beautiful, emotionally charged testimonial and practice description videos.

Honestly, making these videos and watching them after is my very favorite part of our process because it is so intimate, we really get to know our clients, their patients and their shared dreams and idiosyncrasies. We learn what makes them talented, special humans and we share it with the world, more specifically, we share it with potential patients who are looking to make a decision about a fee-based medical or dental procedure.

## Social Media: Mostly Facebook

Facebook CEO Mark Zuckerberg and I are different brands of entrepreneurs, different types of success stories and different types of workers. We have a few things in common though, namely we were both in our 30s before we earned our degrees from Harvard, and we received our diplomas on the same (very rainy) day.

You see, Harvard has a very generous policy for students that allows for long leaves of absence and extended degree completion timelines. So, in a strange turn of events both Mark and I sat through the same soggy commencement ceremony, we both watched Dame Judy Dench and James Earl Jones receive their honorary degrees. As you might imagine, the rain fell unevenly upon us to the extent that my mortarboard and tassel was soaking wet and his was bone dry, such is the seating prioritization of honorary doctorates bestowed to brilliant, billionaire demigods vs. latent undergraduate degrees granted to mortals who are merely "bright" or "promising" by comparison. My diploma got wet and some of the crimson color from its envelope bled onto the parchment, I didn't order a replacement diploma because I thought the effect looked cool and signified the blood that I sweat to get the degree in the first place.

While I usually am the definition of decorum while attending such formal festivities, I did get a self-shot video of me congratulating Mark. He issued a brief "thanks" in my general direction as he walked past me and into Widener Library, but he didn't bother returning my congratulations:

I guess he must have just been star struck to meet me or something.

Anyway, Mark's invention has proven to be pretty key for our Elite 300 clients. In many ways, it's far more important than Google.

Yeah. I know you've heard it before at conferences or have read about it on blogs, *"social is important."* The speakers or authors usually cite the growing number of Millennials who are entering the market with a growing amount of disposable income and that social is generally the way that they prefer to engage new business.

It's true. Millennials do like to use social to learn about new businesses. That's not new information, but what might be enlightening is that Gen X and the Boomers are using social to find and engage new consumer to business relationships as well. The number one mechanism they use to do this is Facebook Messenger.

Facebook Messenger is darn important. The reasons for this follow:

- Facebook is quickly becoming a player as a self-contained search engine. People are searching more now for groups and businesses on Facebook than they ever have. Facebook is not just for connecting people anymore, it's for connecting period.

- Facebook Messenger is super low friction. You pop it open and just message someone. Messenger tells you about how long it has historically taken them to respond and within that amount of time (or sooner) you'll generally get a message back from the business.

- Facebook is its own provider of NAP citations. You see all the contact information, a map and hours-of-operation information, as well as several posts from the business that could show testimonial videos, before and after pictures and current "special offers."

- Facebook Ads that lead directly to the Facebook Page for a client are often cheaper than an ad that sends a user off of Facebook's platform. This is because Facebook is concerned with their "dwell time" also… starting to see a pattern here?

So, we focus mostly on Facebook, but have a program to post on a few other popular social networks as well. In Part IV we will give an overview of a basic Facebook strategy for a practice.

Facebook drives business though. Facebook gets you new patients. It's important to do Facebook (and Instagram) professionally, even if you don't do it privately.

Your competitors either doing it (so you HAVE to do it to compete) or they are not doing it (so you HAVE to do it to dominate).

Either way, all I have to say is again:

*"Congratulations Mark!"*

# CHAPTER 10

## Track Everything

The old joke in marketing is a client that says: *"I know that 50% of my marketing is working, I just don't know which 50%."*

I say "old" joke because it originated decades ago as the result of a combination of radio, television, print and display advertising. These advertising mediums are "dumb" mediums, I use the word "dumb" not in the parlance of our time meaning "stupid" or "unthinking," rather I mean that those forms of advertising are "unable or unwilling to speak."

How do you get data regarding views or conversions (sales) from plastering your face on a bus bench or a billboard? Sure, you can use traffic estimates regarding the number of cars that travel past certain intersections each day, week or month. You can then calculate a certain percentage of persons that would glance up from their gauges at your billboard. A certain percentage of those, one can assume, might have an interest in the medical or dental services that you are selling. A certain percentage of those interested might remember to write down the email or phone number or web address, and a certain percentage of that percentage might even contact your office. A dumb billboard is a crazy way to spend $3,000 a month (or $100,000+ a month in Times Square) and is more about a combination of ego and hope than anything else; as they say, "your ego is not your amigo" and "hope is not a strategy".

You need numbers. Only by relentlessly reviewing fresh, contextual and relevant numbers can you gain true insight into the return-on-investment (ROI) for your marketing dollars. Only then can you intelligently scale your marketing efforts.

## The Sole Metric: Top Line Revenue

Have you ever heard the term of art: "If you can't dazzle them with brilliance, baffle them with bullshit?" Most Internet marketers will use complicated analytics dashboards full of colorful graphs and charts that show the number of clicks and the number of visits per page and it all looks quite exciting. DigitalGoals obviously has the ability to generate some pretty sexy reports, but there's really only one metric that truly matters to our Elite 300 clients, can you guess what it is?

Top line revenue growth.

That's it. That's all that matters from a marketing perspective. Bottom line numbers have too much black magic in them to control with addbacks for car leases, air travel, doctor-owner draws etc.

Don't buy into a spiky-haired Internet marketers technobabble about "audience awareness saturation" or "brand evangelization" these terms only really matter for national consumer packaged goods brands like General Mills, Frito-Lay or Coca-Cola. They want to penetrate the subconscious of the average grocery shopper who is wide eyed in the snack aisle of the local super market to get them to try their specific combination of sugar and carbs or carbs and salt to hopefully get them and their lovely family addicted to the taste.

This type of advertising doesn't work well for doctors and dentists, except in what we call our Authority Ramp program which is part of the "Patients for Life" strategy.

In 2020 and beyond, doctors and dentists will see patient

growth from two areas: word of mouth via citation-based-star-reviews (Google, Facebook, Yelp) and Google / Facebook pay-per-click (PPC) advertising.

So, while we can give you a shiny-happy-report full of colored bubbles and pie charts, we find that our Elite 300 clients (who are doctors just like you) prefer a simple spreadsheet that focuses on just a few areas:

- Total Dollars Spent
- Total New Patients
- Total New Reviews
- Total New Prospects Phone Calls
- Total New Prospect-To-Patient Conversions
- Total Organic Non-Phone Inquiries (form submissions / chat / FB Messenger)
- Total Paid Non-Phone Inquiries (form submissions / chat / FB Messenger)
- Cost per Lead (Phone + Non-Phone)
- Cost per New Patient
- Average Revenue per Patient (Mean / Median / Mode)

That's it. You don't need anything else. Input and output. Simple. All of the graphics and charts in the world isn't going to make those numbers different for better or for worse.

We add those up at the end of every month, then at the end of every year and figure out if our decisions have been directionally correct and whether or not to pour gas on the fire or stamp it out completely.

As of the publishing of this book in November 2019, we haven't had an Elite 300 client cancel a contract with us yet.

In the spirit of full transparency, I will say that these metrics are FAR simpler to collect, tally and report if a client has trusted us to outsource their entire sales process from marketing to actually closing the patient via telephone. **This option seems expensive when you look at the sticker price, but once you realize that you can cut some front office salaries and increase sales... it really should pay for itself.**

## Data Collection: 3 Key Methods

There are three primary methods of data collection that we use for our simple tracking spreadsheet:

1. Dynamic Call Tracking
2. Pay Per Click Tracking
3. Organic Search Engine Optimization Tracking

Even though we tend to present data in a very simple spreadsheet we still do use the very sophisticated tracking methods on the back-end because we do actually use the pretty graphs and charts to fine tune the data that we manually populate the simple spreadsheet with. Let's talk a little about each of the methods:

### Dynamic Call Tracking

When most doctors think about "clicks" they don't immediately think about a phone call; however, they are some of the best clicks a doc can ask for? Why? Because a click-to-call on a mobile device means that a potential patient liked the idea of your offering so much that they are calling for more information or to make an appointment. There isn't a lead hotter than this kind of lead. These are the leads that we hunt like a pride of hungry lions, focusing to generate more than 50% of our Elite 300 clients' leads as click-to-call per month.

How do we do this? We use artificial intelligence (AI) to track specific keywords from prospective patients who inquire about your services via phone. It works like this:

1. We generate unique phone numbers for your practice
2. We assign specific numbers to:
   a. Facebook Ads
   b. Google Ads
   c. Your Website
      i. The website actually has multiple numbers that it assigns to visitors as they roam from procedure area to procedure area so we can understand what they are most interested in when they call your practice
3. We place PPC ads with Facebook and Google to drive calls
4. When the calls come in, we record them using our HIPAA compliant technology and data storage system.
5. After the calls are recorded, the system processes the data and the artificial intelligence engine will highlight key phrases that we consider to be important top-line-revenue-drivers for the practice such as:
   a. Breast Augmentation
   b. Invisalign
   c. Rhinoplasty
   d. Laser Whitening
   e. Full Arch Replacement
   f. Joint Injections

   Or anything else that we decide would drive massive top-line revenue to your locations. I say locations because you might have different offices in different cities that specialize in different procedures as some of our Elite 300 clients do.

6. We collect the data at the end of the month and mine the data for follow-up calls to be made by the practice to close deals that may have slipped through the cracks.
7. Finally, we categorize the call into one of a five different categories
   a. Existing Patient Call

  b. Non-Lead Call (vendor, employee personal call, etc.)
  c. New Prospect (booked appointment)
  d. New Prospect (did not book appointment)
  e. Missed Call

This granularity is so important, especially when used to keep one's own practice employees honest and help them improve their phone game. Not only that, but now you can't be fooled by a spiky-haired-Internet-marketer into thinking that you have received more lead calls than you actually have. An aggressive percentage of new-patient calls should be around 25% of the total calls received. Can you imagine if every fourth time the phone rang, your office manager could be signing up a new patient?

Imagine, now we can see the metrics coming from the ad source (Facebook / Google) and, in some instances, align that with a specific person who has called your practice! <u>That's powerful accountability for your marketing dollar.</u> Again, when we know what works… we can scale it.

**Pay Per Click (PPC) Tracking**

I was having lunch with a partner that I have in real-estate ventures at one of his two beach hotels last month.

I initially met him at his $30 million spec-house that he built to sell to a hedge fund manager. He held the Harvard Club "Welcome Back" party there where he made the point to tell all of us that he was a high-school dropout.

After selling a few hundred million dollars annually in real estate annually and building multiple hotels and other luxury properties his wealth exceeded anyone's in the room and might have been close to the aggregate of the other total members (there were only a couple dozen members invited).

Mr. Nicholas Shawn Chavez

While I can't be sure, I imagine this was a very proud moment for him; to be, for a moment in time, the envy of a group of individuals who routinely think themselves a part of the elite.

I liked him. A lot. We chatted a bit at the party as he gave a highlights-only tour of the nearly 30,000 square foot home to my wife Jes and I. I flattered myself into thinking that I saw many similarities between he and myself and I wanted to learn more about him.

At the follow-up lunch I asked him if he thought it might be easy to sell that massive beach house. He indicated that it was all about putting it in front of the right set of eyes.

Then I blew his mind.

I told him that we could use Facebook Ads to target the occupants of a single building in NYC that held multiple billionaire residents. I explained to him the method by which we target Facebook users for our Elite 300 clients and by the end of lunch, we had decided to explore doing business together for his expensive properties.

My focus is doctors of course, but the principles for marketing a $30 million beach house are the same as marketing a $25,000 medical or dental procedure. Anyway, I told him that I didn't want him to pay me a monthly fee, but that I wanted a percentage of the transactions I set up; like when we represent a medical or dental practice for sale[13].

He liked that we could track billionaire prospects using some of the same tools and technologies that we use to track prospective patients for doctors.

Google ads and Facebook ads are a great start to get people into the sales funnel. *Now believe it or not, it's actually easier to adver-*

*tise to billionaires as potential buyers for a $30 million beach house than it is to market to your existing patient base.*

Why? Because HIPAA, that's why.

One spikey-haired-Internet-consultant was daft enough to write in his book the illegal / unethical advice to "upload the email addresses and phone numbers"[14] of your current patient base to Facebook so you can "clone" your Facebook Audience.

**Damn man. That is SO dumb.**

He just put his entire readership at potential risk in the name of saving or generating a few bucks for their practices through Facebook marketing. His clients might get slapped with HIPAA violation fines and jail time, and he bears the risk of that also.

**What an awful way for those doctors to potentially lose their practices and reputations and everything they've worked their entire adult life for.**

Anyway, we can make Facebook Ads and Google Ads work for you without violating HIPAA or HITECH. We build the ads based upon keywords, geography and the demographics of the audience that you are looking to address. Depending upon how specialized this data is, and whether you are targeting the billionaire inhabitants of a single building or simply the wealthiest 10% of users in a certain zip code… your ads may cost a lot or a little.

The cost per ad shouldn't be your primary concern, rather, you should be thinking about ratios. Let's think about the math for a moment, consider these scenarios:

- If you bought an ad for $1 and could generate $1 in profit, would you buy the ad?

- If an ad cost $500 per click but could generate $600 in profit, would you buy the ad?

- If an ad cost $750 per click but could generate $3,000 in profit, would you buy the ad?

In reality, all of these ads are amazing buys. The price tag might be shocking at first, but as long as the metrics back it as a profitable play, why wouldn't you buy the ad? Actually, the only question you should be asking yourself after you've evaluated the veracity of the data is "how many ads like this can I buy before the market is saturated and they stop working?"

This is digital marketing at scale. Even with the first ad being essentially break-even, have you analyzed the lifetime value (LTV) of the patient? Maybe the break-even is only in Month 1, and in Months 2-100 the patient generates more revenue to make sure he or she is a profitable client.

The lesson here is that if the PPC campaign is operating at break-even or better, it's a keeper. This is easier said than done, but once you get there… it's pretty sweet.

## Organic Search Engine Optimization Tracking

Search Engine Optimization (SEO) is a black-bag operation and I wish to hell it wasn't.

I wish Google would just come out with a user manual illustrating how to simply optimize a web site for inclusion onto the top three results of the first page of Google results. They obviously do NOT do this, and the reason why can be understood in the examination of the differences between a *rating system* and a *ranking system*.

I'll use a story from earlier in my career to simplify it:

IBM is a ~$100 billion technology company, one where I've worked twice; once prior to graduating high school and the other prior to graduating college. As someone that had returned to work at IBM, I was considered a "boomerang" hire and during my second tour I was significantly more senior in terms of salary and title than my first tour; but the annual review system was largely the same.

IBM had a *rating system* for their employees that also served as a *ranking system*. The rating system was easy enough for people to understand and it was organized as 1 (best) through 4 (worst), but the ranking system told a different story:

- 1: To be ranked as a "1" was the highest honor one could receive in his or her review, my wife Jes who also worked at IBM was ranked as a 1. In addition to her being smarter than I am, people generally liked her better also. 1s received the highest salary bumps and were first in line for promotion.

  A competency / practice area had a handful of these to spread around amongst many dozens, if not a hundred or more employees. Generally, 1s represented 2-5% of the total.

- 2+: This is where I was ranked, not because I didn't deserve a 1 rating, but because politics being what they are in senior management, I wasn't as close with my manager as the two people in my practice who were ranked as 1s.

  He explained that there were only "so many 1s that could be given out" due to the allocation and that I "definitely deserved" to be rated as a 1.

  I was pretty bitter about this, especially when I found out that the guy who was given the "1" rank took his promotion to Partner and leveraged it into an offer as a Managing Director for Deloitte. Evidently, he and my manager worked together in Houston many years prior, or at least so I was told.

This mis-applied rank of 2+ was lucky though: Had they graded me a 1 and made me a Partner, I would have stayed at IBM, with its blue blood running through my veins... probably until I reached retirement age. Looking back at it, that would have been a major step down from what I do now in terms of mission satisfaction and aggregate potential compensation.

Employees ranked 2+ represents the top 6-10% of IBMers.

- 2: Employees ranked as a "2" generally show some leadership qualities that allow their managers to give them more responsibility and authority. 2s being somewhat common, they are a mobilized class that tends to receive the majority of the promotions, though perhaps not as quickly as a 1 or a 2+.

2s represent the top 11-20% of IBMers.

- 3: This is essentially average. 3s did their jobs satisfactorily and would continue to be paid and receive marginal pay increases and promotions every few years if there was a vacancy they could fill. 60-70% of IBMers fall into this rank.

- 4: These people are on their way out. They are not meeting expectations in one area or another. They are one restructuring away from being jobless, in the worst instances they are simply fired due to incompetence or an improper "culture fit" which could mean a great number of things, but most often everyone assumed it meant that the person was an ass.

Why talk about IBM's ranking system? Well, *ranking systems* have to do with real-life constraints whereas *rating systems* do not.

You see, if there were no rewards / resources tied to annual reviews, then it wouldn't be important to force rankings… one could give ratings as they saw fit and could fudge them a bit higher to ensure everyone "felt good" and continued to have a high morale.

Given that money is limited and so are promotion spots, the "rating system" translates into "rankings".

This is the same for search engine results. There can only be one first result on the first page for any given term, right? That's why SEO is so competitive and constant, there are only 10 Results displayed on every standard Google search results page (very few users change their preferences to get up to 100 results per page) so given that there are only 10 results on page one for any given search term, Google keeps the criteria to rank as a highly guarded secret on par with KFC's original recipe, the formula for Coca-Cola Classic and POTUS' launch codes.

The other maddening part about this is, that Google changes their ranking algorithm regularly… sometimes as often as multiple times per day. So, a page-one ranking today may not mean a page-one ranking tomorrow… and the old joke goes: *"Where's the best place to hide a dead body? The second page of Google results."*

So, with SEO, very few organizations can get it right. We even miss the mark sometimes for our Elite 300 clients who are paying considerable dollars for our expertise. Luckily, we've done a pretty good job explaining to them that SEO is a moving target.

We have found that there are three areas that move the needle for organic SEO:

1. Excellent content, written in sufficient quantity
2. Proper metadata hooks for written, image and video contents
3. Citation replication and proliferation

From a tracking perspective, we make a massive effort to ensure that we track important keywords and phrases for our doctors and dentists and the results show. For every patient we bring for our doctors organically, that's one less click that they have to pay for.

It's awesome. We will go over the mechanics in depth in Part IV for those of you who either cannot afford to hire DigitalGoals, or if you just have a high tolerance for the pain associated with reading dull quasi-technical language.

# PART III: ACQUISITIONS

*Price is what you pay. Value is what you get.*

Warren Buffett

This is going to be a fairly quick overview of M&A for local medical and dental practices. We will give you the broad strokes of the numbers that you should look for when buying (or selling) your practice as well as some of the mechanics that you will need for the transaction. Essentially, every single deal is different and therefore will need special advisory; however, there are commonalities that can be addressed in a quick framework.

Per my earlier description of what DigitalGoals does and does not do; we may advise our Elite 300 cohort members regarding an acquisition, a merger or a divestiture but we may or may not choose to take a fee for doing so.

Whether or not we take a fee will depend upon the following decision matrix:

1. Is our Elite 300 client comfortable with DigitalGoals taking a fee?

2. Have we truly earned the right to take a fee in addition to the monthly fee that we have billed the client; meaning, did we do anything extraordinary to cause this introduction or did it occur as the result of work that we have already been paid to do?

3. Is there already a business / transition broker in the deal? We love partners, mostly because they insulate our doctors with additional expertise. We will defer fee to these

experts if they are necessary to get a deal closed in a less-risky way.

As you can see, we default to "ethics first." Our business is designed around long-term relationships, not around a sole transaction or even a handful of transactions. So, we will defer-fee and choose to work with an acquisition team that is comprised of:

- A medical / dental practice accounting specialist
- A medical / dental practice acquisition attorney
- A medical / dental practice transition broker
- A medical / dental practice transition banker

We can and will help select these professionals for our Elite 300 cohort members. We go out of our way to network with these professionals and they have offered to send business our way also, should they identify an elite doctor in need of Internet Marketing.

It's a pretty good system.

## CHAPTER 11

## Growing Via Acquisition

When you establish or buy the first location of your dental or medical practice, you are essentially purchasing a job for yourself.

In some cases, this job is very stable and is fairly lucrative. For some, this is quite satisfactory, and they want nothing more than to enjoy their middle-to-upper-middle-class income and fish, hike, surf or binge watch the latest Netflix Original on their days off. That's a nice, relaxed life. I'm happy for them.

To others, this isn't enough. Some doctors crave luxury appointments and a significant amount of leisure time to pair with their increased disposable income and the fun things or experiences it affords. Very few single-location doctors reach any level of what we could call true "wealth," as such, we must figure out how to scale a practice. The first and most obvious way is to hire associates and support staff for your primary location, the second is clearly to replicate the success that you've experienced with your first practice location. The best part is, the location you buy might well be more successful than the practice that you currently own and run.

Since the economics for specialist physicians and dentists are so different, the advice given also changes. We will give sample data for both doctors and physicians so, depending upon which kind of doctor you are, you'll have a great idea of what you might want to be looking for and about how much you'll want to pay to acquire satellite practices. For now, let's focus on a few commonalities.

## Finding Practices to Buy

Just like anything, this takes hustle and network.

You didn't really think that you could just ring a broker up on the phone and tell her you were ready to buy a dental or medical practice, did you?

Furthermore, how many calls like that do you assume she gets in a week? How many of those calls are already pre-qualified to buy a practice with a bank and the appropriate down payment?

Brokers can be tough people to deal with, simply because they are well practiced in the art of protecting their time from dreamers who don't have the dollars, advisors or the requisite plan to execute a deal.

Literally THE most important decision that you can make associated with this is the quality of life that you are looking to achieve, and the "must-haves" associated with your career.

For the purposes of this book; I am going to assume that you are running an existing practice and you are looking to expand your local footprint. It's what we teach at DigitalGoals, because ideally we have expanded your patient throughput for your current location to or near your absolute maximum capacity and the only way to grow is to start knocking down adjoining walls and building your existing office out or buy a competing office in or near your geographic location.

Before you start looking for a practice, you need to know answers to the following questions COLD:

- What is your annual production for each of the last three years? What is the average?

- What are your collections percentages for each of the last three years? What is the average?

- How much cash do you have to deploy toward the practice purchase? (You generally need around 10% of the purchase price in cash or a minimum of around $50-75k.)

- What is your credit score (should be around 700) and your debt-to-income ratio based upon the income amount that you and your practice reported on taxes last year?

- How soon are you looking to pull the trigger on a practice?
  - Immediately
  - 1-3 Months
  - 4-6 Months
  - 7-12 Months

- Will you allow the current doctor to stay in the practice as an earn out and for how long?

Having answers to these questions will impress brokers, bankers and attorneys who can help you source practices to buy. Know that if you are an Elite 300 cohort member and Digital Goals client, we will have already surveyed with you the local competitive market, so you'll have some options with which to go forward.

We can also introduce attorneys, accountants and bankers.

## Checking Financials

Any practice that you are considering for acquisition should have a well-documented history of cash flow. This serves two purposes:

1. You are better off starting with patients than without patients.

2. You should have a decent idea of what the practice's per-patient-revenue is, how much money the practice is collecting and what the accounts receivable aging looks like.

Essentially, you'll be looking very closely at the percentage of collections and what the selling doctor is taking home as his or her percentage of personal production or percentage of personal + associate production.

In order to get this information, you'll need to examine the Profit and Loss Statement (P&L) of the target practice that you are looking to acquire; you'll then want to ensure that the numbers from the P&L report match the tax returns for the practice over the months and years that make up the examination period.

Let's cover a few important expense categories that you'll want to keep a close eye out for when you are reviewing a P&L for a practice that you are looking to buy:

- Employee Costs (around 25%-30% of collections)
  - Salaries
  - Payroll Taxes
  - 401k match
  - Holiday Bonuses
  - Continuing Education

- Lab Supply / Services (7.5%-15%)

- Real Estate Mortgage / Rent (7.5% - 15%)

The margins of a healthy practice should be somewhere around 30-45% after you have "added back" the doctor's BMW lease payment, salary and any other expenses that he or she is taking out of the practice. Remember to reconcile these numbers with the practice tax return.

## Of Entities and Taxes

I dislike talking about taxes as much as I dislike talking about accounting (because I am not an accountant); but you need to know this stuff. Obviously, check with a real accountant about this.

Most practices are organized as either an S-Corp or an LLC that files as an S-Corp. In the event that this is not the entity structure, it will generally be either a partnership (LLP) or a professional corporation (PC); you'll want to inquire of your accountant to understand the differences between these, but for now let's stick with the S-Corp / LLC example.

You'll be reviewing their 1120S which is the tax return for either of these structures used in most U.S. states. You may also be looking at the practice owner's Schedule C, which generally means that the practice is not being ran as an S-Corp or LLC.

I will not go so far as to steer you away from Schedule C practices that are generally sole proprietorships because the profitability of the practice can be hidden in all of the Schedule C deductions.

Unfortunately, there really isn't a hard-and-fast rule regarding this analysis. It's case by case.

We will take a look at the legal structure and the numbers with you; but your accountant and attorney should give you guidance with finality.

## Letters of Intent

Letters of Intent (LOIs) for a practice purchase are simultaneously a very important part of the acquisition process and often non-binding, which is to say that they are not worth the paper that they are printed on.

There is a lot of psychology that is happening at this point in the process, most of which is rooted in persuasion, greed and fear. It's one of my favorite activities in which to engage because most of the logic that was present in the due diligence phase goes right out the window.

Most doctors, and humans in general lose their marbles when they are looking at a big number that they are either going to pay or receive as payment.

My advice here is to make this part of the process as personal as possible. Send the LOI to the seller with a handwritten thank you card and cement the personal relationship that you have embarked upon during the due diligence phase. Your attorney should ensure that all parties are receiving this document simultaneously so there is no room for anyone to unilaterally change the terms.

There are two sellers in this phase. The seller of the practice, and the buyer who is selling the seller as to why they are the right doctor to buy the practice and at what price.

## Your Teammates

We've talked at length about how to identify a good coach and why having one is important; but we haven't talked much about the teammates that you'll want on your side of the ball in order to successfully buy or sell a practice.

If you are an Elite 300 cohort member, we will be the cornerstone of your team and may not even charge you a fee for helping to quarterback your acquisition. The other members of your team are not going to give you "free" fees because your relationship with them will often be classified as "transactional" as opposed to "ongoing" except in certain negotiations with your attorney and accountant.

**Attorney**

I received a few scholarships to law school, and I still may someday attend; though, I cannot imagine going back to the freezing cold northeast for another three-year tour at another Ivy League school. The curriculum at most law schools (especially for the first year or what is referred to as "1L") is nearly identical due to the standards set forth by the American Bar Association (ABA). So, I think I'll choose my law school, should I make the decision to go, based upon proximity to loved ones or a nice beach.

I digress.

The point is, that the market for legal has become as commoditized as medicine if not more so. The competition for legal work has exploded along with corresponding increases in enrollments for law school.

So, many of these dental / medical transition attorneys will work for a flat-fee as opposed to an hourly bill rate.

You probably want the flat-fee attorneys, unless you are recommended to an hourly attorney that has done good work for a reasonable price.

All in, you really shouldn't be paying this attorney more than around $10k. If it is much more, or much less (by 20-30%) you might be prone to worry a bit, again, unless the attorney has come through a referral from us at DigitalGoals or another source that you trust.

To ease your mind, we refuse all referral fees from attorneys. We look at them as a conflict of interest (but we might let them buy us a beer or a steak as a thank-you.)

## Accountant

God bless accountants. They have, in my opinion, one of the most difficult jobs in the world. I do not say this because of the math involved. I like math. I'm good at math.

The difference is that for all the math that I've ever done, the numbers are already there for me. Accountants need to hunt down the numbers, infer or generally deal with missing information all the time and they have to be comfortable with issuing opinions around it.

For a very short time I had a job working in an accounting department for a Fortune 1000 company. The position was as a Director of Financial Systems and Process, where I was in control of all of the systems that calculated the accounting that would report numbers to Wall Street for that publicly traded company. The crux of the issue was that I was a Director-level employee and sat in a nice golf-course-view office next to another Director-level employee who had been at the company for a number of years.

He was a forensic accountant and would often spend his lunches in my office alternatively marveling and laughing about the way that our company auditors (one of the very, very big firms) would sign off on our financials without really understanding the cross-company accounting for related transactions.

I hated the idea of being in control of the systems that were processing the accounting that may be somehow misreported. According to my accountant-colleague, there were several irregularities that he reported to senior management and the auditors where nothing was ever changed.

I begged to be reassigned. No luck. My boss was a foreigner that had naturalized as a U.S. Citizen and his name was on all of the Securities and Exchange Commission (SEC) filings as well. Little did I know that he was planning his exit from the company also.

He and I didn't like each other much.

I was given a form from the auditors that I was to sign stating that I did not see anything that would be flagged as irregular for Sarbanes Oxley (SOX). I told my boss I wouldn't sign it. He insisted. I pushed back.

I won the first round by begging off since I had not been there for a full quarter by the time the form needed to be signed. That didn't work at the end of the second quarter.

Instead of signing the form, I documented on the form all of the information that my colleague had told me and given it to Internal Audit, who launched an investigation.

To his credit, the CFO of the company (my boss' boss) asked me into his office and sat me down to thank me for my diligence. The General Counsel also sat down with me in an attempt to allay my fears.

Still, I was very uncomfortable and made that point very clear to everyone who would listen. As you might imagine, my boss was pretty irritated with me at this point and his irritation manifested through repeated texts at 9-10pm when I was still in the office asking me why I took a bit of personal time around 3-4pm earlier that day.

I suppose the math might have been a bit difficult for him, but at the time of his repeated texts had already put in around 11 hours for that day (which was not altogether uncommon).

That was it. I quit the next day and I haven't thought about that boss since; though, I have kept in touch with a few friends from the company and sent an email explaining my reasons for quitting to the Chairman and another to the CFO. Neither of them responded.

My former boss left for an executive position at a regional accounting firm no more than two weeks after I quit. I mention this to remind you to make sure you check your accountant's background closely. Just because an accountant has a CPA and a fancy title doesn't mean that they are ethical or a good fit for your practice.

**If you just skipped to the last line of the accounting section, I don't blame you. Accounting is hard and boring. The moral of the story is:**

*Don't use the other doctor's accountant. Get your own and make sure that he or she is a GOOD one that specializes in medical or dental practice transitions.*

**Banker**

Kristina is a classmate of mine from Harvard; we had the great fortune of having Dr. Peter Marber as our professor for our Emerging Markets class while he was also portfolio manager for emerging markets at Loomis, Sayles & Co. He's since left to run the Aperture New World Opportunities fund which is benchmarked against the Bloomberg Barclays EM USD Aggregate 1-5 Year Total Return Index. He's also written a handful of books about economics and emerging markets. If you are looking for an educational beach read in the field of economics, I recommend any of them whole-heartedly.

I mention Dr. Marber simply because he has a high standard for excellence, one that I ostensibly hit after achieving an A-minus in his class; but someone else who was hit that standard was Kristina, who at the time was participating in the class as part of a Graduate Certificate in Corporate Finance.

When Kristina and I met for rooftop drinks at the Harvard Club in NYC after our class; she asked how we might work with one another. I considered a few possibilities outside of her managing my money (I choose to do so on my own); and it hit me:

"Does Bank of America Merrill Lynch have a department that works with doctors and dentists to help them finance new practices?" I asked.

She was right with me. She indicated that BofA did have a department that handled loans for doctors and dentists (as well as a great many other services) and she introduced me to Ken, John and Jason who work with *Bank of America Practice Solutions*.

**I should say right up front that I am not compensated by BofA or any of its employees for recommending them here or by sending referrals their way.**

Before you start looking for an angle, I'll just admit to it:

I will refer doctors to BofA simply because I like connecting good people with other good people, and the less money doctors and dentists spend on interest and banking fees, the more money they have to deploy into marketing to ramp up their revenue.

Now, I am not saying that you should blindly go with BofA. I'll say that you should strongly consider making them one of two choices; with the other bank being whomever else has been referred to you in good stead (ask your aforementioned accountant or attorney for a recommendation).

A little bit of competition is good between banks; but don't fall into the trap of sourcing a handful or more bankers from different banks; the attention might feel good for a while, but you will invariably irritate one or more and those can be counted as bridges burnt.

We all have finite time, so it's best not to waste your own or that of others. Be respectful of their expertise, profession its inherent limitations.

Medical and dental practice transition is a very small world indeed.

Anyway, for the hard and fast numbers that I know some of you will be looking for, here are some estimates. Your rates and loan limits will vary depending upon your creditworthiness, your production / collection ratio, the production / collection ratio of the practice you are looking to buy and the underlying interest rate environment that is prevalent in the market at the time you are looking to borrow the funds.

- Minimum Loan Amount is $250,000
- Maximum Loan Amount is $5 million
- Interest Rates 2.99% - 8%+

Beyond the banker analyzing your personal production and creditworthiness you'll also need to need to work with the banker to complete a Site Analysis and together make a decision whether it's best to finance the entire amount of the practice or less. A good banker will also work with you to help you understand whether you should take an interest-only loan or one where you are paying down principal.

Your coach, accountant and attorney can help you a bit with these calculations as well but trust me when I say that you're going to want to pick a banker you like also. You'll need them again when it's time to yet-again buy another practice.

## Business Broker

When I was a bit younger and had a fair amount of arrogance that had not yet been counterbalanced by wisdom, I thought of most brokers as thick-headed, lazy individuals who didn't care much for hard work, hard-math or penning complete sentences.

Like a great many other opinions I held in my youthful verve, this too was incorrect. The key element that I was ignoring was that brokers weren't simple order takers; the best ones were merchants of the most important commodity in the world: information.

Let's put this into context:

Let's say that you are looking for a lake house in which to spend vacations on Tahoe with your family and friends. You plan to celebrate birthdays there, you plan to erect a two-story Christmas tree in the living room and you plan to buy a shiny chrome Weber grill so you can survey the lake from your deck as you cook dinner for your crazy children and their screaming, laughing crazy children.

But, you can't find this house.

None of the houses that you have looked at are *quite* right; maybe the home has a deck, but without a lake view, maybe it has a living room, but not one that will accommodate your considerable holiday décor vision, maybe the floorplan isn't open enough for everyone to enjoy watching your grandkids demolish their 1-year-old birthday cake. Who doesn't want to see blue frosting smeared all over a laughing cherub?

Does this perfect vision of a house just not exist on the market? You checked the MLS, Zillow, Redfin, Trulia and every other electronic realty site you could find. No luck.

It's out there. A broker knows about it, but it's not on the market yet. They have a name for these, they're called:

*Pocket listings.*

Essentially, a homeowner will have seen a well-known broker at a local bar or the bait shop, and they'll catch up a bit. After the idle chatter, the owner will hint that she is looking to sell her two-story, open floorplan, lake-view home but she isn't quite sure and doesn't want to go through the "bother" of listing it and having it shown if the probability is low that the house will sell. Afterall, she doesn't want nosey neighbors peeking through her stuff in an open house.

The real estate broker keeps the unofficial listing in his "pocket" and makes a mental list of buyers who may be interested in the home and discreetly contacts them indicating that the house "may" be for sale if they or a friend of theirs might be interested in buying.

Get it? Good.

That exact same process happens for medical and dental practices somewhere in our fine country EVERY SINGLE WEEK. It's even more private though, because the presiding doctor is generally also the owner of the practice and she is NOT going to risk scaring her patients away by putting a big "MY PRACTICE IS FOR SALE" sign out in front of the parking lot.

A good practice transition broker will have an intimate knowledge of local practices that want to merge, buy or sell.

The market is consolidating, you need all the big brains you can find on your side or you'll be working for another doctor, one you'll call "boss."

**Coach**

We've been through this in detail; but I wanted to take a quick moment to remind you that you absolutely NEED a good coach; this is not some fluffy elective that you can just skip over so long as you have some Tony Robbins audiobooks and a pot of strong coffee.

You need someone who has "been there" before and someone who understands practice economics and the ins-and-outs of practice transition.

Even better, if you have someone who is involved in your monthly business who can advise on your situation specifically because they understand your revenue creation model and your expense structure.

Again, DigitalGoals may not charge additional for this work, so it can be good to use us AND a specific coach. We don't know everything, and often the coach doesn't either; but working together, you can go into your practice purchase or sale knowing fully well that you have folks looking out for your best interest who will guide you before, during and after the transition.

## PART IV: EVERYTHING ELSE YOU NEVER WANTED TO KNOW ABOUT INTERNET MARKETING

*A wise man can learn more from a foolish question than a fool can learn from a wise answer.*

Bruce Lee

# CHAPTER 12

# Who Not How

One of my mentors in the Internet Marketing space taught me to ask a very important question: "Who?" not "How?" As a result of this being drilled into my head, I've asked him to contribute some technical learnings to this book for practice owners who could not afford to hire an Internet marketing company and I have normalized his writings to apply to practice management for doctors and dentists.

## Once Upon a Time Near Washington D.C.

There were no markings on the gate that provided entry through the ten-foot-tall black security fence. Should you be daring or silly enough to scale this fence, there isn't razor wire at the top, rather each "pale" or bar in the fence is bent outward and sharpened like the tip of a hunting knife. We were entering the premises of a data center critical to the global economy.

Inside the gate, the grounds were beautifully landscaped with lush greenery and a lovely pond. I was later told that the pond was installed to create a hard, 90-degree angle in the road to prevent someone escaping with valuable data. Once inside the facility we were shown through anonymous white hallways into a nerve center where less than 80 people have access, inclusive of military, employees and contractors. Within this area are servers developed by IBM that cost $20 million each, rooms full of oversized car batteries that can sustain the servers for up to 48 minutes in the case of an outage until one of a dozen house-sized diesel generators can get to full power and run the servers for weeks, months or years if the electric-grid was truly offline for that long. Interestingly, it only takes 30 seconds for all of the generators to get to full power, far less than the 48 minutes the batteries could sustain the servers.

Onsite was a post-office facility that received all incoming mail and packages. If a package was received that was somehow tainted or deemed dangerous to the data center, the foundation of the post-office facility could detach, and the ENTIRE POST-OFFICE could be airlifted away from the data center.

The architects built in redundancy after redundancy. I was in awe.

I'd like to think that I could design something like that. I want to believe that I could; but I probably couldn't. Despite my past involvement in U.S. Government systems and facilities there is absolutely NO WAY I could have designed something that intricate. After spending a bit of time at that facility as well as similar facilities for CISA and NSA I remembered something that my Google mentor from South Florida taught me:

> Train yourself to ask WHO not HOW. HOW is a blank-check in terms of your money and your time but asking WHO gets you to the root of exactly how long it will take and how much it will cost.

I never forgot that. You see, I have a true belief in my innate ability to do almost ANYTHING. Outside of playing any type of professional sport, I truly believe that I could train myself to do anything well. I always looked at this as a strength, but I realize that it is a weakness in one very real way: it creates MASSIVE opportunity cost.

Not to mention: why the hell would I want to design a high security data center anyway?

I realize now that I can do ANYTHING but I can't do EVERYTHING. As a graduate of medical or dental school, I imagine that your brain has a similar capacity. You tell yourself that you can do anything, and you likely could train yourself to do so… but we all only have 24 hours in a day, so you MUST prioritize your interests and your actions. You must do what you do best to bring in the most money or enjoyment into your life.

The issue is, you can only really be ultra-selective with your time and interests if you already have money, either in assets that can be liquidated or in the form of a high-income. Either can be redistributed for the purpose of employing people to do things you COULD do but have decided that the opportunity cost is too high.

**WARNING: THE REST OF PART IV IS FOR DOCTORS WHO HAVE A PRACTICE THAT IS GENERATING $500K OR LESS.**

### Part IV Overview

Part IV is specifically designed for the doctors and dentists that are just now coming out of medical or dental school, and don't have the revenue-generating-practice necessary to become one of our Elite 300 client doctors. In the spirit of "who not how" I have asked my friend and mentor to supply some of his best teachings for Part IV of the book.

So, to all of the new docs who have six figures in student loans and the energy to stay up all night to put the magic of the Internet to work for you; please find some detail-oriented guidance that was given to me by my friend and edited specifically for your consumption and application.

Could a doctor take this information and give it to a low-level employee to do on their own? Possibly; but I am near-certain that they won't be as effective or cost efficient as DigitalGoals in doing so.

Put it this way, if you can afford to pay an employee to do this poorly, you can afford to pay DigitalGoals to do it well. If you can't afford it, and you need help then let's get started.

**Throughout Part IV, we will lay the foundation to map out your online marketing plan:**

- A basic plan for your practice Facebook page

- Your online marketing plan (Website, SEO, PPC, Pay-Per-Lead services, etc.)

- Start with the fundamentals (Market, Message, Media) before jumping head first into your Internet marketing strategy

- How to setup your website

- Understand how search engines work and learn the differences between the paid, organic and map listings

- Search Engine Optimization - How to optimize your website with keywords that are most important for your particular business

  ◦ How to conduct Keyword Research
  ◦ Our list of the most commonly searched keywords broken down by industry (Dental, Medical, Plastic Surgery, etc.)
  ◦ How to achieve maximum result by mapping out the pages that should be included on your website
  ◦ How to optimize your website for ranking in the organic listings on major Search Engines
  ◦ How to improve your website's visibility so that you can rank on page one for your most important keywords
  ◦ List of link building techniques and strategies that are

proven to enhance rankings even in the post Penguin and Panda Era
- Content marketing strategies for maintaining relevance in your market

- Google Maps Optimization - How to get ranked on the Google Map in your area

  - The fundamentals of Google Maps ranking (NAP, Citations, Consistency and Reviews)
  - How to establish a strong Name, Address, and Phone Number Profile
  - How to properly claim and optimize your Google+ Local Listing and merge it with Google Places, if necessary
  - How to merge your Google Places and Google+ Local listing if you have a preexisting Google Places account
  - How to develop authority for your map listing via Citation Development
  - List of the top citation sources for medical and dental practices
  - How to get real reviews from your customers in your true service area

    - Sample Review Card
    - Sample Review Request Email
    - Sample Review Us landing page for your website

- Website Conversion Fundamentals - How to ensure that your website converts visitors into leads in the form of calls and web submissions

- Mobile Optimization - How to optimize your website for mobile visitors

- Social Media Marketing - How to utilize Social Media

(Facebook, Twitter, Google+, LinkedIn and other social platforms for maximum effect in your dental or medical practice

- Video Marketing - How to tap into the POWER of YouTube and other video sharing websites to enhance your visibility and drive better conversion

- Leverage email marketing tools (Constant Contact, Mail Chimp, etc.) to connect with your customers on a deeper level, receive more reviews, get more social media connections and ultimately get repeat and referral business

- Overview of Paid Online Advertising opportunities

- Pay-Per-Click Marketing (Google AdWords and Bing Search) - How to maximize the profitability of your Pay-Per-Click Marketing efforts

  - Why PPC should be part of your overall online marketing strategy
  - Why most PPC campaigns fail
  - Understanding the Google AdWords Auction process
  - How to configure and manage your Pay-Per-Click campaign for maximum ROI

- Paid Online Directories - What paid online directories should you consider advertising in (Angie's List, YP.com, Yelp.com, Judy's Book, Merchant Circle, etc.)

- Pay-Per-Lead and Lead Services - How to properly manage Pay-Per-lead services for maximum return and long term gains

  - Sample lead follow up email sequence

- Track, Measure and Quantify - How to track your online

marketing plan to ensure that your investment is generating a strong return

When it comes to Internet marketing for your practice there are a number of avenues to explore. In this chapter, we will briefly touch on the various Internet marketing channels that are available, and then go into more detail throughout the book. This chapter serves as your "Marketing Plan" and roadmap going forward.

**Online Marketing Channels**

1. Search Engine Optimization (Organic Listings and Map Listings)
2. Search Engine Marketing/PPC on Google AdWords and Bing Search Network
3. Social Media Marketing (Facebook, Twitter, Google+, LinkedIn)
4. Video Marketing
5. Email Marketing
6. Paid Directory Marketing (Angie's List, Yelp, etc.)
7. Paid Lead Services

Proper application of the above will build a framework that looks like this:

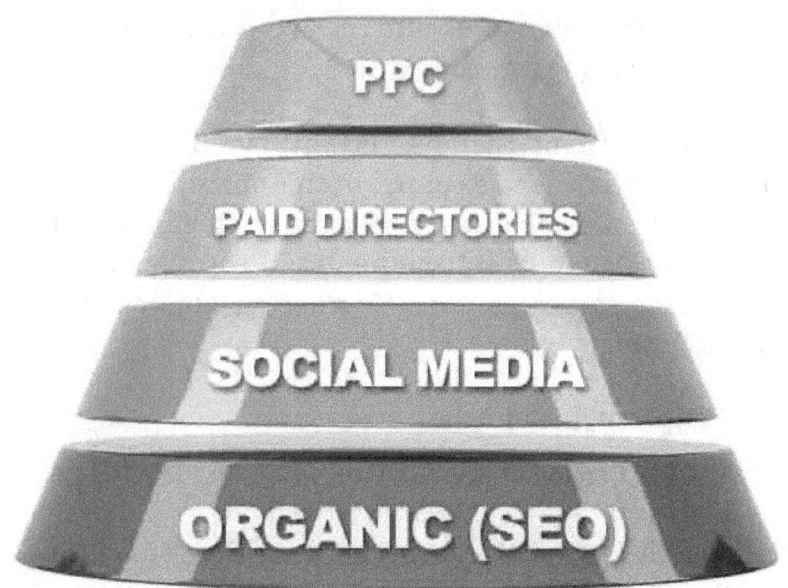

## Search Engine Optimization

Search Engine Optimization (SEO) is the process of increasing your practice's visibility on major search engines (Google, Yahoo, Bing, etc.) in the organic, non-paid listings as patients are searching for your products or services.

There are three very critical components of Search Engine Marketing. The three components are:

- Paid Listings – The area along the top and side where doctors can bid on and pay for in order to obtain decent placement in the search engines.

- Organic Listings – The area in the body of the Search Engine Results page.

- Map Listings – These are the listings that come up beneath the paid listings and above the organic listings in a number of searches.

Search Engine Optimization involves getting your website to show up in the Organic and Map Listings. These listings account for a majority of the search volume. As depicted in the illustration below, more than 78% of searchers click on the Organic (non-paid listings) rather than the paid listings.

When most people think "Internet Marketing," they think Search Engine Optimization. However, you will begin to see that SEO is only a small piece of the MUCH BIGGER "Internet Marketing" puzzle for doctors.

**Search Engine Marketing / PPC**

Now that we have discussed SEO, let's talk about Search Engine Marketing or PPC (Pay-Per-Click). Google, Yahoo and Bing all have paid programs that allow you to BUY listings associated with your keywords to be placed in designated areas of their sites.

There are three really important benefits of PPC:

- Your keyword listings will appear on search engines almost immediately.

- You only have to pay when some actually clicks on your listing – hence the term Pay-Per-Click Marketing.

- You can get your ad to show up on national terms in the areas/cites in which you operate.

PPC Marketing works on an Auction system similar to that of eBay. You simply choose your keywords and propose a bid of what you would be willing to pay for each click. There are a number of factors that determine placement which will be discussed in detail in the PPC for Doctors chapter. But, in the broadest sense, the doctor who is willing to pay the most per click will be rewarded the top position in the search engines, while the second-most will be in the second position, etc.

PPC Marketing is a great way to get your company's website to appear at the top of the search engines right away, driving qualified traffic to your website.

**Social Media Marketing**

There is a lot of BUZZ around Social Media (Facebook, Twitter, LinkedIn, YouTube), but how can it be utilized by a doctor? How can you use social media to grow your practice?

- More than a billion active users
- 50% of our active users log-on to Facebook on any given day
- Average user has 130 connections
- People spend over 700 billion minutes per month on Facebook

So, how can you employ this amazing tool to grow your practice? Use it to connect with your personal sphere of influence, past and new patients. By doing so, you can solidify and maintain existing relationships, remain Top-Of-Mind and ultimately Increase Repeat and Referral Business.

**Video Marketing**

Did you know that YouTube is the second-most used search engine on the market? Would you guess that it is ahead of Bing and Yahoo? It's true! Millions of people conduct YouTube searches on a daily basis. Most doctors are so focused on SEO that they completely neglect the opportunities that video and YouTube provide. By implementing a Video Marketing Strategy for your business, you can get additional placement in search results for your keywords, enhance the effectiveness of your SEO efforts and improve visitor conversion.

**Email Marketing**

Similar to Social Media Marketing, Email Marketing is a great way to remain top-of-mind with your customers and increase repeat business and referrals. Compared to direct mail and newsletters, email marketing is by far the most cost-effective means to communicate with your customers.

As we will discuss in the Email Marketing for Doctors chapter, we feel that email marketing can be used to effectively draw your customers into your social media world.

**Paid Directory Marketing**

There are a number of Online Directories that are important for doctors:

1. Angie's List
2. YP.com
3. Judy's Book
4. City Search
5. Merchant Circle
6. Yelp

**Paid Lead Service sites**

There are an array of services that will sell you leads on a "pay-per-lead" basis or a flat monthly fee. I don't think any of them are good. They usually sell the same lead to 3-4 different doctors or dentists, so usually the first doc to call will get the patient, that is IF the prospective patient is serious enough to make a decision.

**WHERE TO START?**

With such a large number of Internet marketing channels, where should you start? I firmly believe that over time, you should be appropriating each of these online marketing opportunities. However, you must first begin with the foundation - your website, organic rankings and social media/email. You should start looking at the various paid marketing opportunities when your website is setup correctly, ranking on search engines for your most important keywords in the organic, non-paid listings and you are actively engaging in social media activity. We have found that the biggest and most impactful opportunity is getting ranked organically (in the non-paid listings). You may then leverage the additional profits in paid marketing to further augment your growth. Once you are ranking well organically and things are firing on all cylinders, then you can start to run a well-managed Pay-Per-Click Campaign and explore paid online directory listings.

Next, let's look at the fundamentals of your overall marketing strategy before pressing forward into full implementation.

## Start With Fundamentals

Before we delve into Internet marketing, SEO and social media marketing, I want to be sure we have built a strong marketing foundation. As I talk with medical students across the United States, I have come to the realization that the vast majority of them tend to skip straight past the fundamentals of a practice marketing strategy and dive head-first into tactics (Pay-per-click advertising, SEO, Social Media, etc.).

So, what do I mean when I say "Fundamentals"? All marketing has 3 core components:

1. Message (what)
2. Market (who)
3. Media (how)

You have to have a unique "message" (who you are, what you do, what makes you unique, and why someone should hire you rather than a different doctor), a specifically defined "market" (who you serve to and who your BEST patients are), and THEN look at "media" (where you can reach those BEST patients). The advertising tactics (Pay-Per-Click, SEO, Social Media, Direct Mail, etc.) fall into the "media" category.

If you focus solely on media or tactics, you will likely fail regardless of how well-selected that media is. With that being said, you need to scale back to the fundamentals. You need to invest the time and energy in fleshing out your "message" and figuring out who your "market" is; and by doing so, all of your "media" choices will be vastly more effective. Make sense?

Good, now spend a few minutes and THINK. Take out a scratch pad and answer these questions:

**Message:**

- What do I do that is unique and different from my competitors?

    - Do you offer a guaranteed time frame for your appointments so patients don't need to wait in the waiting room?
    - Do you offer free initial consultations prior to starting the procedure and promise to stand by that estimate?
    - Maybe you offer a guarantee for all of your work and will remedy any issues within a one-year period of time after the procedure is complete?

- If you think about the psychology of a patient, what concerns or apprehensions do you think they have about hiring a doctor?

    - *"They won't see me on time, so I will probably have to waste the whole day waiting around for them..."*
    - *"They are going to talk over my head in medical language I don't understand and think I'm stupid..."*

- *"They are going to give me one price over the phone, tell me another when they get me into their office and then charge me something VASTLY different once all is said and done."*

- How can you address your patients' common concerns in a unique way?

**Market:**

- Who is my ideal customer? (Please realize that geography isn't as much a factor as it was in years past. Get more specific than "Everyone who resides in my city or within a 25 mile radius of my office."

- Take a look at your last 25 procedures and evaluate who spent the most money, who had the highest profit margins and who was genuinely pleased with your service.
    - What are the unique characteristics of those good patients?
    - Are they home owners vs. renters?
    - Do they live in a particular area of town?
    - Do they have a higher income level?

- Start to define who your ideal customer is so that you can put a marketing plan in place to attract similar patients.

Once you have fleshed out your message and your market you can start to think about media. In order to determine what media will be most effective for you, you need to think about where you can reach your IDEAL patient.

**Media:**

Clearly, the Internet is a great "media" for connecting with your ideal patient who is proactively in the market for your services.

Throughout the remainder of this book, we will be explaining the various Internet marketing channels and how you can use them to connect with your ideal patients.

Please remember, you need to start with the FUNDAMENTALS (Message, Market and Media) before running headstrong into any marketing endeavor.

Don't put the cart before the horse. It is expensive and futile for your practice.

## CHAPTER 13

## How to Setup Your Own Website

This chapter is all about how to setup your website. You shouldn't be doing this by yourself, but if you are just starting out in medicine and don't have the cash to hire someone, you need a solid reference.

Later in Part IV, we will eventually cover details as they relate to SEO, Google Maps Optimization, Pay-Per-Click Marketing, and the like; however, without a properly designed and functioning website, those efforts amount to little more that wasted time and money.

Before you begin exploring those options, you must have your website up and running. Let's talk about website formats and the different options that are available to you when you are ready to start.

1. HTML Site – There are basic HTML pages and/or individual pages that can be incorporated into a website. This is how almost all websites were built several years ago with multiple pages hyper-linked together manually. Some of these custom sites were beautiful to look at, but could take 6-9 months to build out properly due to the necessary coding.

2. Template Based Site Builders - Site builders, that you can obtain through providers such as WiX, Weebly and Squarespace are close to turn-key products. Essentially, you buy your domain and set up your website in a few hours. The simplicity of these services are outweighed by

the inflexibility and lack of control a practice has with these options; not to mention the idea that Google's algorithms do not like templated sites with stock content (images or words). So, this is certainly an option of last resort for a practice that needs to stand out in a commoditized medical or dental marketplace.

3. CMS Systems - Content Management Systems, like WordPress, Joomla, Drupal and MotoCMS that will create a framework around custom content to be input into the practice's site.

We have proven that a content management system is ideal for your practice. The reason that I say that is because you have scalability. In any of these platforms, you have the ability to change your navigation on the fly, add as many pages as you need and easily scale out your site. If you have your website built in WiX or Website Tonight or in HTML format with graphics behind the website, and you wanted to add a new section, you would have to start from scratch. You would have to go back to the graphics and modify all of the pages in order to add the new section to your navigational structure. With a CMS, everything is built behind code allowing the ability to apply easy edits and to add multiple pages.

As you will see in the search engine optimization section of the book, you will have the ability to have a page for each one of your services and each city that you operate in.

A CMS allows you to create your pages in a scalable format without having to mess around with the graphics or do anything that is difficult to control. Also, it is easy to access, modify, and update. Using formats like WordPress and Joomla, you may access the back-end administrative area at *yourcompany.com/login* or similar.

After entering your username and password, you will find that there is a very easy to edit system with pages and posts that function similarly to Microsoft Word. You can input text, import images and press "save," forcing all new edits to be updated on your live website.

Content Management Systems have intelligently structured linking between pages and content, making it extremely search engine friendly. We have found that this method tends to be better than regular HTML or WiX type options. In a lot of cases, a blog is going to be automatically bolted onto a CMS based website providing you with a section where you may feed updates. In the SEO chapter, we cover the importance of creating consistent updates and blogging regularly.

Another benefit of a content management system is that you are provided with a variety of plugins or widgets that you can choose to incorporate on your website.

- You can easily pull in your social media feeds, YouTube Videos and check-ins.

- You may also syndicate your website to automatically post any new updates to your social media profiles.

- You can add map integration where people can click to either get instructions or view a heat map from where your patients are requesting service.

- There are a surplus of features available within a CMS that you can't necessarily do with a non-CMS type option.

Whether you are looking to build a website from the ground up, if you are just getting started, or you feel like you simply need a redesign, I highly suggest that you do so in a content management system: ideally in WordPress or MotoCMS. WordPress is a fantastic platform and very easy to use. It's the most adopted website platform available with a lot of developers working on it. It's constantly being updated and improved and I have found it to work very well for medical and dental practices.

## Navigation

So, what features should your website have? What navigation structure should you create?

You definitely want to have:

1. Home
2. About Us
3. Our Services
4. Our Service Area (You will understand what I mean once you read the SEO Chapter)
5. Online Specials or Coupons
6. Reviews and Testimonials
7. Before and After photos of procedures
8. Patient Guide
9. Blog
10. Contact Us

These are the core pages. Within "About Us," you might incorporate a drop-down menu for subcategories including "Meet the Team," "Why Choose Our Practice," etc.

These can be very powerful ways to connect with prospective patients.

## Give Them a Reason to Choose Your Practice

Most people will read your site before choosing you as their doctor, so it's extremely important that you infuse personality into your website in the form of authentic photos and videos.

Mr. Nicholas Shawn Chavez

Don't use stock photography, instead use custom authentic imagery.

Showcase your company, feature yourself, the practice owner as well as the people that work in the business: the nurses, hygienists, technicians and the front office team. Showcase your office itself, the waiting room and the surgery operatories as well as the newer, specialized equipment if you have any.

This gives the visitor the chance to get to know, like and trust you, before they even pick up the phone. I've seen this tactic prove itself time and time again.

For example, let's say a potential patient visited two different practice sites:

1. A site with an image he or she has seen before of the same generic doctor with his plain white coat, stethoscope and a weird smile. No video, just a wall of text to get through with fake doctors and nurses holding their thumbs up.

    OR

2. An authentic, genuine site with a picture of the ACTUAL primary doctor, videos of the team, the waiting room and equipment.

The authentic page converts visitors to patients 10 to 1 over the generic site. You must let your real personality reflect on your site.

Further, it is important to craft messaging that explains why a prospective patient should choose your practice. Help them understand why they should choose you over another doctor who may be closer or charge less per procedure. Define a narrative that explains why you are their best option by providing social proof in the form of online reviews and potentially make use of some special offers and incentives that will drive them to visit your practice for the initial consultation. This simple combination of social proof and incentives drives them to contact your practice right away, as opposed to continuing to browse the web for another doctor who performs similar procedures.

## Describe Your Services and Service Areas

Within "Our Services," you want to have the ability to list a drop down menu listing the types of services and procedures that you offer. Also, you'll want to have landing pages for each one of your services because they are going to be optimized for Google searches through the use of different search-keyword combinations.

A "Service Area" section will give you the ability to show a heat map of all of the nearby cities and towns that your practice services, as well as a drop down menu that lists the sub-cities within your market.

## Reviews and Testimonials Are Important

A "Reviews and Testimonials" page will provide you with a section to showcase what your customers are saying about you in text or video form. You can also pull in reviews from sites such as Google Maps, Angie's List, and Yelp.

You should also post your credentials either in the sidebar or in the header graphic, proving, for example, that you're BBB-accredited or a member of the local chamber of commerce or industry association. This allows potential customers to rest assured that you are a credible organization, that you're involved in the community and that you're less apt to provide them with poor service. They'll feel more comfortable doing business with you.

## Make it EASY for Them to Contact You

Know that not every visitor to your website will be in a similar online environment. Some may already be on their phone dialing around contacting doctors in the area about procedures; and luckily, this type of prospective patient can simply pick up the phone and call you; however, someone may not have the ability to stop what they are doing and make a phone call to your practice without drawing unwanted attention from his or her coworkers. This is why it is important to enable quick and easy ways to browse around your website to find out what procedure options and pricing charts are available.

You will need a "Contact Us" page where web visitors have your general contact information.

In addition to the Contact Us page, you should always provide your primary phone number on every page of your website, in either the upper or lower right-hand corner. So, when somebody visits a page, their eyes are naturally drawn to the top section of the website, the logo and the phone number. This is practice is rapidly becoming industry standard, so prospective patients tend to expect that phone number will be somewhere in this location.

Company name, address and phone number on nearly every page of your website is non-negotiable. It is not critical that you list your address on each page because it will not be a determining factor in whether or not they call you, but as I will explain in the Google Maps optimization section, having name, address and phone number consistency is critical for ranking on the Google Map

One way to accomplish this consistency is to have your name, address and phone number referenced on your website, ideally in the footer section. You need to have that contact information on all of your pages including the Contact Us page, of course.

In any scenario, your potential patients must have a simple, no-pressure way to enter their information into a web form where they can provide their name, phone number, email address, and a note detailing their situation.

In addition to the contact details, you also want to provide links to your social media profiles. Link to Facebook, Twitter, Instagram and LinkedIn so customers can easily engage with your practice on social media and press the "Like," "Follow" or "Subscribe" button.

## Is Your Website Mobile-Ready?

The other major thing you want to think about, from the conversion perspective, is having a mobile-ready version of your website. More and more people are accessing the Internet via smart phones such as iPhones and Androids. You need to make sure that the mobile version of your site isn't the same as your regular site. It should be condensed, fitting their screen and giving them just the information that they need. It should integrate with their phone so all they have to do is press a button to call you. People that are searching or accessing your website from a mobile device are in a different state of mind than the people that are browsing and finding you on a computer.

Make it easy for them to get the information they need and to get in touch with you.

## CHAPTER 14

## Understanding HOW Search Engines Work

In this section, we wanted to take a few minutes to demystify the search engines and break down the anatomy of the Search Engine Results Page. By understanding how each component works, you can formulate a strategy to maximize your results.

There are three core components of the Search Engines Results page:

1. Paid/PPC Listings
2. Map Listings
3. Organic Listings

1. **Paid/PPC Listings** – In the paid section of the search engines you are able to select keywords that are relevant to your business, and then pay to be listed amongst the search results. The reason it is referred to as PPC or Pay-Per-Click is because rather than paying a flat monthly or daily fee for placement, you simply pay each time someone clicks on the link.

2. **Map Listings** – The map listings have become very important because they are the first things that comes up in search results for most locally based searches. If someone searches "Vasectomy Reversal + your city," chances are the map listings will be the first thing they look at.

   Unlike the paid section of the search engine, you can't buy your way into the Map Listings. You have to earn it. Once you do, there is no per-click cost associated with being in this section of the search engine.

3. **Organic Listings** – The organic/natural section of the Search Engine Results page appears directly beneath the Map Listings in many local searches but appears directly beneath the Paid Listings in the absence of the Map Listings (the Map Section only shows up in specific local searches).

Similar to the Map Listings, you can't pay your way into this section of the search engines and there is no per-click cost associated with it.

Now that you understand the three major components of the Search Engine Results and the differences between Paid Listings, Map Listings and Organic Listings you might wonder... "What section is the most important?" I know this to be true because it's one of the most common questions we get from our Elite 300 clients when we are having our initial discussions with them.

The fact is that all three components are important, and each should have a place in your online marketing program because you want to show up as often as possible when someone is searching for your specialty services in your area.

With that said, assuming you are operating on a limited budget and need to make each marketing dollar count, you need to focus your investment on the sections that are going to drive the strongest Return On Investment (ROI).

Research indicates that the vast majority of the population looks directly at the Organic and Map Listings when conducting a search, and their eyes simply glance over the Paid Listings.

So, if you are operating on a limited budget and need to get the best bang for your buck, you should obviously start by focusing your efforts on the area that gets the most clicks for your practice at the lowest cost.

*We have found that placement in the Organic and Map section on the Search Engines drive a SIGNIFIGANTLY higher ROI than Pay-Per-Click marketing.*

Begin with the Organic Listings and then, as you increase your profits, you can start to shift those dollars into a proactive Pay-Per-Click marketing effort.

In the next chapter, we will start to look at Search Engine Optimization and how to optimize your practice website to rank in the organic listings (non-paid) for the most important keywords in your field.

## CHAPTER 15

## Search Engine Optimization

Getting your medical or dental practice listed in the organic section (non-paid-listings) of the Google comes down to two core factors:

- Having the proper on-page optimization so that Google knows what you do and the general area that you serve. This allows it to put in the index for the right keywords. You do this by having pages for each of your services and then optimizing them for specific keyword combinations (Ex. Your City + main specialty, Your City + procedure 2, Your City + procedure 3, etc.)

- Creating enough authority and transparency so that Google ranks you on Page One (rather than page ten) for those specific keywords. Ultimately, it comes down to having credible inbound links and citations from other websites to your website and its sub-pages. The doctor who has the most credible inbound links, citations and reviews will be the most successful in obtaining new patients as a result of Google searches.

Throughout the course of this chapter I will provide specific how-to information on exactly what pages to add to your practice website and why. I will also discuss what you can do to improve your authority/transparency in Google's eyes so that your website ranks on Page One for the keywords that are most important to your business.

Before you start creating pages and trying to do the "on-page optimization" work, you need to be clear on the most commonly searched keywords relative to the procedures you offer. By understanding the keywords, you can be sure to optimize your website for the words that will actually drive qualified traffic to your practice's site.

## How to Conduct Keyword Research

There are a number of tools that can be used to conduct keyword research. Some are free of charge and others have a monthly cost associated with them. Some of the better keyword research tools include WordStream, Google AdWords Keyword Tool and SEM Rush.

For the purposes of this book, we have developed instructions based on the free Google AdWords Keyword tool.

- Develop a list of your services and save it in a .txt file

- Develop a list of the cities that you operate in (your primary city of practice and the smaller surrounding towns) and save it in a .txt file

- Go to www.mergewords.com

    - Paste your list of cities in column 1
    - Paste your list of services in column 2
    - Press the "Merge!" button
    - The tool will generate a list of all your services combined with your cities of service

- Go to Google.com and search "Google Keyword Tool" or go directly to *https://adwords.google.com/o/KeywordTool*

    - Paste your list of merged keywords into the "word or phrase" box
    - Press "Submit"

- You will now see a list of each of your keywords with a "search volume" number beside it

- Sort the list from greatest to smallest

You now have a list of the most commonly searched keywords in your area for your medical or dental specialty.

With this list you can map out keywords to specific pages on your website and rest assured that you are basing your strategy on actual metrics instead of estimates.

Based on this data, you will want to create content on your website for the following (sample) keyword combinations based upon high-margin procedures and treatments you provide:

Your City + Doctor
Your City + Surgeon
Your City + Pediatric Dentist
Your City + Dental Veneers
Your City + Breast Augmentation
Your City + Stem Cell Treatment
Your City + Teeth Whitening
Your City + Full Arch Restoration
Your City + Cataract Surgery
Your City + Lasik
Your City + Invisalign

Now these terms are super hard to rank for because there is a TON of competition AND it's hard to write content for your website that is human readable and formatted with proper grammar.

Before you get the wise idea to just SPAM a bunch of keywords and city names on the bottom of your site, know that Google hates it and WILL penalize your site if you try it. They even have a cute phrase for the practice. They call it: "keyword stuffing."

So, what you'll want to do is write content on your page for what is known as "long-tail" searches. So instead of going for "Miami + Plastic Surgeon" you might want to write a blog post titled: "Why women prefer silicone breast implants to saline breast implants in Miami."

See how that gets you where you need to be from a keyword perspective? Google LOVES articles and content like that.

## How to map out the pages on your website for maximum result

Now that you are set to determine the most commonly searched keywords in your field of practice, you can begin mapping out the pages that need to be added to your website.

Keep in mind that each page on your website can only be optimized for 1-2 keyword combinations. If you came up with 25 keywords then you are going to need at least 12 – 15 landing pages (that's a LOT.)

You need to be sure you have each keyword mapped to a specific page on your site.

| Keyword | Mapped to what page |
| --- | --- |
| Main Keyword | Home |
| Keyword 1 | Procedures - Keyword 1 |
| Keyword 2 | Procedures - Keyword 2 |
| Keyword 3 | Procedures - Keyword 3 |
| Keyword 4 | Procedures - Keyword 4 |
| Keyword 5 | Procedures - Keyword 5 |

So, for example, an arthritis clinic in Denver might come up with the following keywords:

arthritis and rheumatology, arthritis dr, Denver doctor, Denver arthritis clinic, Regenexx, osteoarthritis, steroid injections, knee pain

| Keyword | Mapped to what page |
|---|---|
| Denver arthritis | Home Page |
| Denver arthritis Doctor | Home Page |
| Denver knee pain | Knee Pain Treatment |
| Regenexx injections | Injectable Steroids |
| Aurora arthritis | Aurora Arthritis Page |
| Aurora arthritis Doctor | Aurora Practice Page |
| Aurora rheumatology | Aurora Practice Page |

This is just a small sample of what needs to be done. Now that you have mapped out the pages that need to be included on your website, you can start thinking about how to optimize each of those pages for the major search engines (Google, Yahoo and Bing).

## How to Optimize Your Website

### Step 1 – Build the Website and obtain more placeholders on the major search engines.

A typical medical practice website is has only 5-6 pages: (Home – About Us – Procedures – Frequently Asked Questions – Contact Us). That does not create a lot of indexation or placeholders on the major search engines.

Most doctors provide a wide variety of procedures, as covered in the Keyword Research section of this chapter. By building out the website and creating separate pages that highlight each of these procedures that are offered (combined with city modifiers), the doctor can get listed on the search engines for each of those different keyword combinations.

Here is an example:

- Home – About – FAQ – Contact Us
- Sub-pages for each service – Denver Knee Pain, Denver Tennis Elbow, Denver Carpal Tunnel, Denver Regenexx, Denver Arthritis Treatments, ETC

They often provide services in a large number of locations outside of their primary city. In order to be found on the major search engines for EACH of those sub-cities, additional pages need to be created:

- Sub-pages for each sub-city serviced – Boulder Arthritis, Littleton Arthritis, Northglenn Arthritis, Arvada Arthritis

**Step 2 – Optimize Pages for Search Engines:**

Once the pages and sub-pages are built for each of your core procedures, each page need to be optimized from an SEO perspective in order to make the search engines understand what the page is about. Here are some of the most important items that need to be taken care of for on-page search engine optimization:

- Unique Title Tag on each page
- H1 Tag restating that Title Tag on each page
- Images named with primary keywords
- URL containing page keyword
- Anchor Text on each page and built into Footer – <u>Denver Arthritis</u>
- XML Sitemap should be created and submitted to Google Webmaster Tools and Bing Webmaster Tools

# How to Build Authority

Once the pages are built and the "on-page" SEO is complete, the next step is getting inbound links. Everything we have discussed to this point is sort of like laying the groundwork –the pages need to be in order to even be in the running. However, it is the number of QUALITY inbound links and web references to those pages that is going to determine placement.

*30% of SEO is On-Page type work*
*The other 70% is Link Building*

Once the pages are built is just the beginning. The only way to get your site to rank above your competition is by having MORE quality inbound links and citations to your site.

*Doctors who have the MOST quality in-bound links WIN!*

Again, if there is any secret sauce to ranking well in the search engines, it really is links and authority. The major caveat to that is that you can't just use garbage links. You don't want to just have a thousand links. When I say links, I'm referring to other websites hyper-linking to your website, which I'll explain a little bit more with specific examples.

The latest algorithm changes (Google Hawk, Google Core and Google Medic) involve Google trying to prevent spam and look for quality written and video content.

A lot of Internet marketers and SEO coordinators realize it's all about the links. That is what the Google algorithm was built upon. These terrible spikey haired interment marketers figured out methods to get a variety of links with random anchor text pointed back to the pages that they want to have ranked. It's tough work outsmarting Google, who quickly recognized that if links are not relevant to the content of a website then they don't add any value to the Internet and, by extension, to the users of Google.

We talked a bit earlier about Google penalties, and bad or irrelevant links can actually hurt your ranking more than help it. It's about getting quality, relevant links back to your home page and sub-pages through content creation and strategic link-building. How do you get the links? Where do you get the links? Take a look at the visual below as a point of reference:

1. Association Links – Be sure that you have a link to your site from any industry associations that you belong to (Ex. American Medical Association, American Dental Association, Florida Dental Association, etc.

2. Directory Listings – Get your site listed on as many directory type websites as possible (Angie's List, Yahoo Local Directory, Judy's Book, Yelp.com, etc.)

3. Create Interesting Content/Articles about your industry. This is probably the #1 source of inbound links. For example, you can write an article about "incontinence" and push it out to thousands of people through article directory sites that may each contain a link back to a specific page on your site.

4. Competitive Link Acquisition – this is the process of using tools like Raven Tools, SEO Book and others to see what links your top competitors have, and then get those same or similar links pointed back to your website.

**Directory Links** - There's a number of what I like to call "low-hanging fruit" links. It all starts with your online directory listings. Some examples include Google Maps, Yahoo Local, City Search, Yelp.com, Judy's Book, Best of the Web, Yellow Pages, HealthGrades, ZocDoc and the list goes on. All of those online listings let you list your practice name, address, phone number and a link back to your website. Some of them even allow reviews.

For the most part, adding your business information to those directories is completely free of charge. You want to make sure that you have your company listed on as many of the online directory listings as possible for authoritative linking reasons.

They're also valuable from the Google Maps optimization perspective because they give you citations, which are very important for getting ranked on the map. A great way to find additional online directories to add your company to would be to run a search in Google for "Your Practice Type – Business Directory" or "Your City – Business Directory". This will give you a great list of potential directory sites to add your company to. There are also tools for this like BrightLocal or White Spark, that can provide you with a list of directory sources based on your specialty. After beginning with online directory listings, you want to look at any associations that you're involved with.

**Association Links** – Above I reference AMA and ADA. I'm assuming you are involved in some type of association, whether it is the national association, the local chapter or some other group affiliation. Visit the websites of those organizations and get listed in the member section. This will give you citations and the opportunity to link back to your website.

**Affiliated Industries and Local Businesses that are non-competitive**- You can work with colleagues that have affiliated industry type businesses. If you're in dental, go to the dental labs in your area and ask if they will post a link to your website on their own site and vice versa. Utilizing your resources and teaming up with relevant companies will add more authority to your domain name.

**Supplier Sites -** The next thing you could look at is the suppliers that you purchase from. If you are a regular customer at Henry Schein, Johnson and Johnson, Karl Storz or if you've got a co-op agreement with Invisalign or some other manufacturer, try to coordinate a deal with them. Oftentimes, the places where you buy your supplies and equipment will have a section on their website that mentions their medical and dental partners. You can get a link from those.

**Social Media Profile Links** - The other "low-hanging fruit" links are social media profiles. We have a whole chapter about the power of social media and how you can harness it to get repeat and referral business. Simply from a link-building perspective, you should set up a Facebook page, Twitter account, LinkedIn profile, Instagram Feed, Pinterest profile and a YouTube channel and place a link to your website on each. Each one of them will allow you to enter your company's name, address, phone number a description and, of course, a place to put your website address.

**Local Association** - Other local associations that you're involved in. If you're a member of the Chamber of Commerce, a networking group like BNI (Business Networking International), or if you're involved with a local charity, find out if they list their members on their websites. Another great place to get links is by typing in your city directory.

**Competitive Link Acquisition** - You might be surprised that if you really tackle these elements and you don't do any of the other things we have discussed, you will notice that you've probably got enough links to outrank other practices in your area. I want to share some additional thoughts and strategies on how you can accomplish even more from a link building perspective. A very powerful strategy that you can implement is called Competitive Link Acquisition.

The way I like to think of it is: if quantity inbound links are the secret sauce to outranking other docs in your area, and if we could figure out who's linking to those other docs or what links your competition have, and we can get those same or similar links pointed back to your website, then you can outrank them, because you'll at that point have more authority! BOOM!

Competitive link acquisition is the process of figuring out who is in the top position for your most important keywords, reverse engineering their link profile to see what links they have and getting those same or similar links pointed back to your website. A simple way to do this is just to go to Google.com and type in "your city + your specialty," and find out who is in the top few positions. Let's take a look at the number one placeholder. He's there because his website is optimized well and Google knows that he should be ranked well based on the quality and quantity inbound links compared to the competition.

Once you know who he is, you can use a couple of different tools such as Raven Tools, Majestic SEO, Back Link Watch, etc., and you can take their URL, input it into your tool of choice, run the report, and get a list of links in return.

So, your practice's number one competitor is *ohiohappyrheumatology.com*. Google spits out a list showing that they have 392 inbound links.

- The practice has a link from the local Chamber of Commerce.
- The practice has a link from the AMA.
- The practice has a link from an article that the doctor wrote for the local newspaper.
- He's got a link from the local physicians networking chapter.

By analyzing the types of links that he has, you can systematically mimic those links and get them pointed back to your website.

Don't just do this for your first practice competitor, but also for your second and third and fourth and fifth practice competitors. By doing that on a consistent basis, you can start to dominate the search engines for your most important keywords.

If you build out your site for your services and sub-services, optimize the pages using SEO best practices and then systematically obtain inbound links, you will start to DOMINATE the search engines for your procedure related keywords in your area.

**Content Marketing Strategies**

Another highly important factor in SEO is relevant ongoing updates to your website. In the Internet age, content is king.

Google loves fresh content. In some cases, with the changes in the algorithm, just because you've got a great website with the right title tags and all the best links, you may get discounted if they're not seeing fresh information posted on a consistent basis. It is important to have a methodology where you are creating and posting content to your website on a regular basis. I want to give you a framework for figuring out what kind of content you could write, why you should create content, and how you can do it consistently.

First, you need to understand and accept that you need to become a subject matter expert. You might not consider yourself a writer or a content creator, but you ARE a subject matter expert.

You are a DOCTOR. (That's kind of a big deal!)

There are things that you know that the general population does not. You're a surgeon, a dentist or a chiropractor and you have a team of people that are experts in this area as well. You can create content on the topic that you know most about.

You can write about the differences between Ritalin and Adderall, what kind of lasers will stop gum disease in its tracks, or the evils or benefits of Universal Health Care. There are a lot of different topics you can come up with that you can create content about, and since you're a doctor, it's bound to be granted some attention and authority.

You should also consider that content doesn't have to be just written words. It's doesn't have to be just articles. Content can come in a variety of forms. The most popular are going to be articles, photos, videos and audio files. Stop and think about what content creation method works best for you.

We crush it for our Elite 300 clients with video. Go to digital-goals.com to check a few of them out. We know how to rank them, so they appear near the top of YouTube searches also. It's amazing.

Anyway, some people are great writers and that's their strength. Other people like to be on camera. I personally like to create videos. I'm very comfortable creating videos (but you need to write the script for those as well.)

Other people can talk, and they can talk your ear off about whatever topic they are passionate about. You can create content in many different ways. Because it is what I enjoy, I'll use video as an example. A doctor can set up a camera and record herself explaining the differences between getting Botox injections and the benefits of a full face-lift in the same manner that she would explain it to a potential patient.

Now you'll actually have multiple pieces of content. You'll have a video, which can be uploaded to You Tube, Vimeo, Meta Café, etc. That one piece of content can create multiple invaluable links to your practice website.

You can also take that video, save the audio portion of it, and you've got an audio clip. You can upload that audio file to your website and post on other various sites. You can use a transcription service like otter.ai, for instance, where you upload the audio or video file and it is automagically converted to text for free. So, for exactly zero dollars, you'll have a complete article comprised of what you said. Now you've got a piece of content you can post to your blog. You can put it on Medium.com or one of those other article directory sites, which BINGO- gives you another link.

You want to create content on a consistent basis, using the blog on your website as the hub to post it, but then syndicating it to various sources. Syndicating it to article directory sites if it's in text form, and sending it to video sites like Vimeo, Metacafe and YouTube.com if it's in video form. Doing this keeps the content fresh on your website/domain and creates a lot of authority, which is really going to help with the overall ranking of your practice website on the search engines.

You want to make sure you're appropriating each one of these link-building opportunities to maximize your rank-potential in your geographic and practice areas. You might be surprised that medical and dental are highly competitive from a SEO perspective. There are a lot of doctors that want to rank for the same keywords, especially for fee-for-service procedures and many of them have invested heavily in the Internet and in getting themselves ranked higher in the search engines.

Okay, now that you've built out your website, you've optimized it correctly, and you've got an ongoing link-building and content development strategy in place, you want to start looking at Google Maps Optimization and getting ranked on the Google Map.

# CHAPTER 16

# Google Maps Optimization

Here's a quick example of one of our dental practices New Day Dentistry who we have gotten onto the Google Maps box, or what we call the MONEY BOX. ☺

This one is a great example because they are in the money box for a very competitive keyword: CITY + DENTIST.

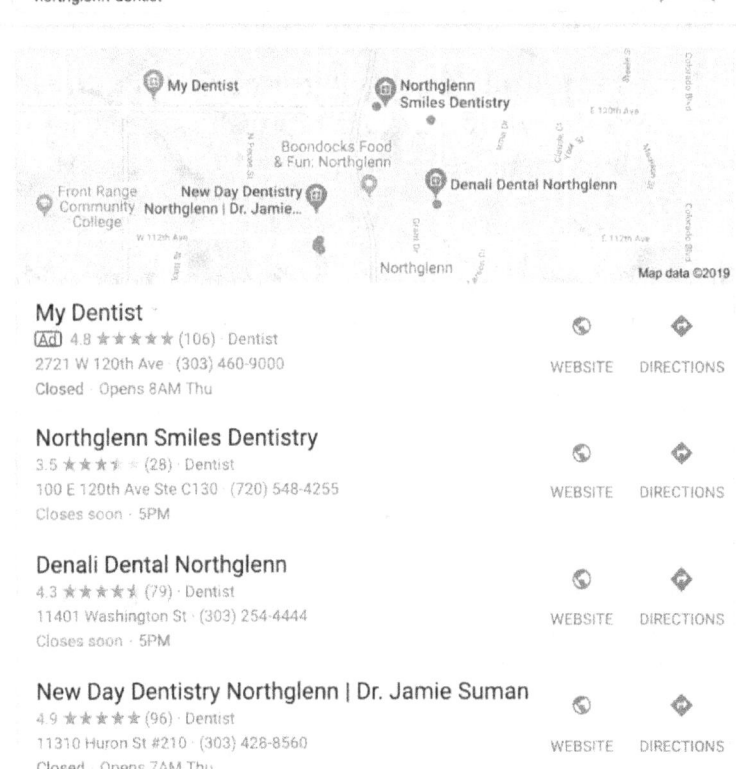

Getting listed on the first page of the Google Map for "Your City + Specialty" comes down to a few primary factors:

- Having a claimed and verified Google Map Listing
- Having a consistent N.A.P. (Name, Address, Phone Number Profile) across the web so that Google feels confident that you are a legitimate organization located in the place you have listed and serving the market you claim to serve.
- Having reviews from your customers in your service area

If you have each of these factors working in your favor you will SIGNIFICANTLY improve the probability of ranking on page one of Google Maps in your market.

## How to Establish a Strong NAP

As I mentioned above, having a consistent Name, Address, Phone Number Profile across the web is essential for ranking well on the Google Map in your area. Google sees it as a signal of authority.

Rather than jumping directly into claiming your Google Map listing and citation-building, it's critical that you start by determining your true N.A.P. so that you can ensure that it is referenced consistently across the web.

When I say making sure that it's consistent, you want to be certain that you are always referencing the legitimate name for your business. If your practice's name is "New Day Dentistry Northglenn", you must always list it as "New Day Dentistry Northglenn," as opposed to just "New Day Dentistry."

The other thing you should be aware of is that there is a lot of misinformation about how to list your company name online. You may read information suggesting that you keyword your name. For example, if your name is "New Day Dentistry," somebody might tell you it would be really smart if you just added to the title of your company "New Day Dentistry | Northglenn Dentist," for instance. While that may have worked back in the day, it's no longer an effective strategy. It's actually a violation of Google Places' policies and procedures. Make sure you list your exact company name the same way across the board on all of your directory sources, you'll see in the example that New Day Dentistry Northglenn has the doctor's name associated with it and a city name. This is okay because it's a single location in a multi-location practice. Google knows this because it's smart and cross references information in the split second it takes to type the search and hit the ENTER button.

**Phone Numbers**

Please make sure that you use the same phone number in all of those places. As we discussed earlier in the book, DigitalGoals is a big advocate for tracking phone numbers and what is happening with your marketing dollars; however, when it comes to your online directory listings, you want to use your primary business phone number that you've been using from the beginning.

Don't try to create some unique number for each one of your directories. What that does is confuses your name/address profile (N.A.P). It will hurt you. Use your primary phone number in all of those places, use your exact company name, and use your principal address, written the same way. If your business is located at "11310 Huron Street, #210," make sure you list it just like that every single time. Don't neglect to include the suite in one place and then put it on in another. Don't spell out "suite" in one place and put "#" in the other. Google and other search engines are looking for consistent name/address profiles across the web.

A good way to figure out what Google considers to be your N.A.P. is to run a search on Google for "Your Company" and see what is being referenced on the Google Map. See how that compares to the other high authority sites like YP.com, Yelp.com, Angie's List and others. Look for the predominant combination of N.A.P. and reference that for all your directory work going forward.

## Best Practices to Optimize Your NAP

- Company Name – Always use your legal Company Name – don't slam additional words into the name field. Ex. If your company name is "Dr. Abrams, M.D.," don't try to put additional keywords like "Dr. Abrams, M.D. Plastic Surgeon in Dallas". This would be against the Google guidelines and will reduce your probability of ranking.

- Address – On the "Address Field" use your EXACT legal address. You want to ensure that you have the same address listed on your Google Places listing as it is on all the other online directory listings like YellowPages.com, CitySearch.com, Yelp.com, etc. The consistency of your N.A.P. (Name, Address, Phone Number Profile) is very important for placement.

- Phone Number – Use a local number (not an 800 number), and make sure it is your real office number rather than a tracking number. We find that 800 numbers don't rank well. If you use a tracking number it won't be consistent with your other online directory listings and will result in poor ranking, so use your main number here.

- Categories – You can use up to five categories, so use ALL five. Be sure to use categories that describe what your practice "is" rather than what it "does". For example, you can use "Medical Center" "Medical Office" and "Medical

Group," in addition to "Plastic Surgeon" and "surgeon".

- Service Area and location settings – Google offers two options here

    1. No, all customers come to my location

    2. Yes, I serve customers at their location.

    As a medical or dental practice you need to select "No, all customers come to my location." because clearly you and your fine staff are not a roving band of Lasik providers who will shoot lasers at people's eyes at their kitchen table. (Unless you are, then call me. I can maybe get you on Oprah.)

- Picture and Video Settings – You can upload up to ten pictures and five videos. Use this opportunity to upload authentic content about your practice. It's always best to use real photos of your team, office, and equipment rather than stock photos.

- Pictures – You can get more juice from this section by saving the images to your hard drive with a naming convention like "your city + doctor – your company name," rather than the standard file name. You can also create geo context for the photos by uploading them to a video sharing site like Panoramio.com (a Google Property) that enables you to Geo Tag your photos to your company's location.

- Videos – Upload VIDEOS. They don't have to be professionally produced (but they SHOULD be, and we can do this FOR you) and will resonate well with your customers. A best practice is to upload the videos to YouTube and then Geo Tag them using the advanced settings.

205

Once you have Optimized your listing using the best practices referenced above, you want to be sure that you don't have any duplicate listings on Google Maps. We have found that even just one or two duplicates can prevent your listing from ranking on page one. In order to identify and merge duplicate listings, run a search on Google for "Practice Name, City".

To clean up duplicates, click on the listing in question and then click "edit business details."

Click "This is a duplicate" to let Google know that the listing should be merged with your primary listing.

If you follow these instructions you will have a well optimized Google Maps listing for your medical or dental practice.

## How to Develop Authority for Your Map Listing Via Citation Development

Now that you have claimed your Google Places Listing and optimized it to its fullest, you need to build authority. Having a well-claimed and optimized Local listing doesn't automatically rank you on page one. Google wants to list the most legitimate and qualified practices first. So, how do they figure out who gets the page one listings? Well, there are a number of determining factors, but one of them is how widely the company is referenced on various online directory sites such as Yellow Pages, City Search, Yelp and others.

Citations are web references to your company name, address and phone number. You can add citations in a variety of ways. There are directory listings that you should claim manually and others that you can submit to via submission services like Universal Business Listing or Yext.com. My personal preference is to claim listings manually, ensuring that I am in control and can make updates/edits as needed.

**TOP Citation Sources to claim manually:**

- Google Local
- Bing Local
- Yahoo Local
- City Search
- Angie's List
- Yelp
- YP.com
- Merchant Circle
- Manta

By securing these high quality citations you will boost your authority and highly improve your probability of ranking in the Google Map Listings. The next critical step is to get online reviews!

## How to Get Online Reviews

The next critical component for getting ranked on the Google Map, after you've claimed and optimized your listing, you've established your N.A.P. and you've developed your citations across the web, is obtaining reviews. You need to have real reviews from your real patients in your true service area.

First, I want to point out that you shouldn't fill the system with fake or fraudulent reviews. You do not want to create bogus accounts and post reviews to Google Map, Yelp, City Search, etc. just for the sake of saying you've got reviews. That's not going to help you. You need real reviews from your actual patients in your true service area.

You might be thinking "Well, how is that important?" or "How would Google know the difference?" Google is paying very close attention to the reviewer's profile.

Mr. Nicholas Shawn Chavez

If somebody is an active Google user and they've got a Gmail account, and they've got a YouTube channel, typically that's all connected to a Google profile.

Say that person with the active profile has had their account for seven years and actually happens to be located in your practice area. If he or she writes you a review, it would be considered credible and will count in your favor. Now, if somebody creates a Google account with the sole intent of writing a review, it obviously is not credible and Google is capable of catching on to that. That account has no history associated with it and it was originated right at your office IP address. That review is going to be flagged as a bogus submission (and you are BUSTED!)

It is important to have an authentic strategy where you are connecting with real people who will write your reviews. You don't want to try and play the system. Google is fully aware, and so is Yelp and a number of other popular online review sites.

With that said, how can you get reviews? What kind of process will you need to actually get reviews from your real patients in your real practice area?

Here's the strategy that we advocate:

> First of all, have some greeting cards printed up. It's basically just a simple card with your practice logo, and a short and sweet thank you note.

"Thanks so much for trusting us with your (procedure). We appreciate the opportunity to serve you as a friend and a patient. We'd love it if you would write us a review." Then give them a link to a page on your website where they can write you a review.

You will want to do some homework on the front end. Be

sure you have a page on your website that is clearly meant for reviews: yourcompany.com/reviews. On that page you'll have links to the various places where people can write your reviews.

We build this into our follow-up management system that we recommend to our Elite 300 practices. It's easy and gets crazy good reviews.

You'll want to have a link to your Google map listing, Yahoo local listing, Angie's List listing, City Search listing and any others that you may have. The reason you want to really have a variety of places where people can write those reviews is two-fold.

Yes, you want to have a lot of reviews on the Google map; but, Google is also looking at the reviews that you have on other websites like Yelp and Angie's List. They're looking at the reviews that you have on Yellow Pages and on Insider pages and on Kudzu.

You need to diversify where you're getting reviews from your customers. It looks more authentic to have 12 on Google, 17 on YP.com and 13 on ZocDoc, than it does if you just have 72 reviews on the Google map.

You want to make it easy and you want to give people options.

The other thing you want to pay bear in mind is that different people use different systems. I am personally a big Google user. If you sent me an email or gave me a card that said, "Please write me a review" and provide me with various options, I'm going to pick Google.

Some people, however, don't have Google accounts. They're not active Google users, but they may be heavily involved in Angie's List or big-time reviewers on Yelp. They're going to have active accounts somewhere. It would be much easier for them to write the reviews where they already have an existing account. The easier and more convenient you make it for people, the better. It's going to bode well in your favor. So, don't try to coax a certain review at a certain site.

Like we mentioned, Google is looking at the reviewer profile. If you only give them one option, and that's the Google map, but they happen to be a Yelp user without a Google account, they would have to go out of their way to create an account to write the review. This is not likely to happen. But, let's say they did decide to create an account. That review is not going to count for much because there's no active profile.

By providing options, the Yelp user that has a reputation for writing reviews and decides to write one for your practice is going to make a difference. That review is going to stick as opposed to being filtered out. Make it easy for them to choose the one that's going to be easiest for them.

Now let's get back to the strategy: Phase One- print out review cards. Have your front office staff hand them out after a service. Have them say something like:

"Hey, thanks for your coming in today! I just want to leave this with you. If you'd be willing to write us a review and share your experience, we would really appreciate it."

It's great. You're showing appreciation. You're holding your practice accountable because you're asking for feedback. By doing that on a consistent basis, you are likely to rack up some solid reviews.

The next thing you'll want to do, just to get a nice little bump in the number of reviews that you have, is to develop an email list of your circle of influence. Your circle of influence is going to be your most recent patients, the patients that have been visiting your practice for quite some time, your family members, and your friends. People that you know, like, and trust who would be willing to act on your behalf.

Put together that email list in an Excel sheet. It might be ten contacts, or it might be 700 contacts. Include the names and email addresses of these folks. Then, use a tool like Constant Contact or MailChimp or another email marketing tool to send an email blast with the following message:

**Email Subject: A quick favor?**

[Name],

I wanted to shoot you a quick email to thank you for the opportunity to serve you as your doctor and to let you know that we appreciate you.

Our goal is to provide 100% customer satisfaction and exceed your expectations every step of the way. I certainly hope that we did just that! If so, it would really help us out if you'd be willing to post a review for us online at one of your favorite online review sites.

Below are a few direct links where you could write a public review about your experience with us:

- **Google** - LINK GOES HERE
- **Yelp** - LINK GOES HERE
- **Angie's List** - LINK GOES HERE

Thank you again! We really appreciate your support!

Best Regards,

Dr. Andrew Corolla

Mr. Nicholas Shawn Chavez

    Tallahassee Facial Perfection

Again, save them the time of having to find the websites on their own by providing some links to the various places to where they can write reviews. By doing sending this email, you're going to create a little bump in your online review profiles. Again, reviews are important. Getting ten reviews on Google Maps is essential. It makes a huge difference in how you rank and it gives you a different perception in the mind of your consumers. You want to get past that 10-review threshold almost immediately.

Doing that helps you get real reviews from real people that have real online profiles. Again, you want to have a systematic process in place where you are asking for reviews on a consistent basis from the patients that you are serving daily. The best way to do that is to request an email address from your patients, either at point of service or after service.

If you move the email ask to the front of the patient interaction where somebody calls in and says, "Hey I need to schedule an appointment, I have a massive toothache." You can respond, "We can get you in right away. Let me gather your information." This is the perfect time to get the email address. Typically, you get their name, address, and the phone number. Well, you can just add one more step at that point and request an email address as well. You can tell them that it is so you can send a confirmation. That's how you start to develop a database of emails. We are going to talk about email marketing later in the book as part of your online marketing plan, but for this purpose, you need an email address so that you can send a message after service thanking them for their business and asking them to write you a review.

The number of reviews that you have from actual patients is going to increase exponentially if you repeat this process regularly. This is how you are going to start to really dominate the Google Map, because reviews and citations work in harmony for ranking.

Remember, we have a system and a software to automate this review collection from your ACTUAL patients (yes, even the old ones).

If you follow these steps to properly claim your Google Map listing, develop your authority via citation development and put a systematic process in place to get real reviews from your real customers in your true service area, you will be well on your way to dominating the Google Map listings in your market for your medical or dental practice.

## CHAPTER 17

## Website Conversion Fundamentals

This chapter is all about website conversion fundamentals; specifically you will learn how to setup your practice website, how to write the content on your website and how to structure the navigational flow of your website to ensure maximum visitor-to-patient conversion.

All of this is intended to translate into increasing revenue you're your practice. Nothing else matters. We target a 300% increase in practice revenue for our Elite 300 clients.

Your results may vary.

I say this because you can have the best Pay-Per-Click (PPC) campaign, search engine optimization (SEO), and be ranked number one on the Google Map, but if your content sucks and the structure of your website isn't set up in such a way that will compel prospective patients to choose your practice over the competition, the clicks won't translate into revenue.

So let's talk about how we can take the traffic we're going to get from the SEO and PPC strategies to push prospective patients to your website that is illustrating a message that will turn these prospects into paying patients.

Here's the key: Be real.

Patients resonate with real people. They want to see their doctor as a real person, in the video content that we produce for our Elite 300 clients, we ask questions like:

*"Where are we most likely to find you on a Sunday morning?"*

*"Are you a Denver Broncos fan?"*

*"When did you know that you wanted to go to dental school?"*

Patients love this. It simulates a friendly conversation over a cup of coffee or a beer.

They like to see the company, the people that they are going to be talking with on the phone and that are going to be going out to their home.

Let the other doctors in your town use the ridiculously posed stock photography. It's hollow, patients as consumers KNOW it. It doesn't connect.

Actual photos, candid (but properly produced) videos and crisp writing really draw people in and it gets them to form a personal connection with the real people who work at the practice.

They see them as real people, and real people are who we all want to deal with. Think about it. If you were to go to buy a new Range Rover, or Mercedes, would you go to the dealership that had stock pictures of the cars and a picture of the dealership building? Or would you prefer to go to a dealership that took a walk-around video of the ACTUAL car you were interested in, started it up to hear the engine note and opened up the door so you could see the color of the interior and the woodgrain of the trim?

You don't sell Range Rovers and Mercedes, you sell yourself and your brilliant mind and skilled hands.

So, for the content of your website craft messaging that draws patients in and makes them connect. They're looking for a doctor that they can trust, so when they land on your homepage, the first message they see should enforce the fact that they can trust you. You should write something along the lines of, "Are you looking for a friendly doctor that you can trust? Then you've come to the right place. Our practice has been operating on the same principles for the last 12 years: trust, value, and excellence." (Or something like that.)

Connect with them! Give them reasons to choose you and have a call-to-action, "Give us a call at this number for an immediate appointment," or, "Click here to take advantage of our online specials and discounts." Remember, they've browsed around the Internet and have seen that there are dozens of practices that they can choose from.

Consider giving them some compelling information about who you are and why they would want to choose you as their doc. Ask them to call now for an appointment, and then draw them into a section where they can get an special offer or some kind of new patient discount. This will incentivize them to choose your practice and make the call ASAP.

When it comes to the written copy on the website, you want to address their specific concerns. On the home page, write something generic, "Looking for a doctor that really knows about _____?" On the procedure page, sympathize with them. "I know how frustrating it can be when you need a specialist and you can't get an appointment. You need to make sure that your health is a priority. We can quickly get you into the office and calm your mind about your situation and come up with a game plan to get you where you we think you need to go."

Write that kind of messaging for each one of the pages on your website including a clear call to action after every block of text saying, "Call now to schedule your appointment," or, "Click here to for an online coupons to get a discount on your first procedure." Pull them deeper into your website with "About Us" links, special offers, and links to before-and-after images, especially for the "WOW FACTOR" type of visuals like teeth whitening, breast implants, tummy tucks, full arch replacements and anti-aging type stuff.

Give them content that makes them think, "these docs know what they're doing," and draw them deeper and deeper into the website so they're more inclined to take the next step. Tell them why they should choose you over the competition. I talked about this in the Message-Market-Media section.

You should also, of course, have a web-form on each of the pages of your website or, at a minimum, on the "Contact Us" page. This is so that if they can't pick up a phone, they can simply type in their name, email address, and phone number and let you contact them.

*Again, make sure that you've got your phone number on the top right-hand corner. You've got a clear call to action telling them what to do next on every page of your website, under every block of text.*

Record a few videos:

- Check out our reviews!
- Download a coupon!
- Look at our before-and-after photos!

Explain why they should choose you. Leverage your personality and hard-won expertise. Be authentic. Integrate your ORIGINAL photos into your website. It really, really helps with conversion.

Utilize your reviews, testimonials and videos. There's no reason you can't create a simple video for each of the pages on your website, explaining what your procedures are, and why you and your practice are the very best at performing them.

Some people are visual, they can see the content on the website, read it and feel fine. Other people are more audible and would prefer to hear the message. If you can spend the time to provide both text and video, it really helps with conversion. Give them external proof. Take them out to the review sites where they can preview testimonials on Angie's List, Google Maps, etc. Or simply embed the results on their pages.

Show them what other patients are saying, and you're going to significantly improve your conversion.

## Example of a Dental Site That is Built to Convert

Internet marketing involves a lot of little things that are performed in sequence to get people to call your company when they are in need of medical or dental attention.

At the end of the month, it all comes down to the amount of calls you received and how much business was booked, right?

1. Company logo should always be in the top left-hand side of the page. The logo shouldn't be overly large. Sometimes clients tell me they want their logo to be triple normal size. The reality is that few searchers know you from your company name, so occupying too much space with just your logo is a waste of valuable webpage real estate.

2. Your phone number is obviously pretty darn important, because very few clients book appointments via web. Your phone number should be as close to the top right-hand corner as possible. Make sure it's large and easy to find.

    Try not to make your prospective patients search for it. It's frustrating for patients and you have just a few seconds to catch their attention before they may move on to another website. Studies show that people always look to the top of the page for that vital piece of info.

3. Professionally shot photos and videos. Have a professional photographer and videographer come in and do their thing. You will use them everywhere. DIY photos and videos are better than nothing, but professional image work is so much better.

4. A small blurb of text talking about your practice differentiators (whether it be that your practice is family-owned and operated for three generations, or that you have the newfangled fountain-of-youth gadget) really brings it all together.

   People buy from people, not cold, boring sterile medical practices.

   Personalize your practice website as much as possible. Your website is your primary marketing tool and it's job is lead capture and to demolish as many buying barriers as possible.

5. Your website's main navigation should be easy to find and the links should be clearly descriptive. Give people the option of moving around your website. One of Google's algorithms is how many pages a person visits and what their visit length was. Guide them down a path without confusing them. In other words, give them all the information they need in as few clicks as possible, but provide them the option of navigating around your site.

6. Some people want a way to contact you without calling. A contact form above the fold (the top half of the page) is great for capturing clients' info. In the case of some doctors, they get a lot of form submissions on a monthly

basis. Without the form, those clients may not have even contacted them. It's also a great tool for building a contact list for email marketing down the road.

7. With your main page content, get to the point right away without going into too much detail. The first paragraph of your text should give you a brief introduction of who you are as a doc and what your practice specialty is. You can go into further detail on your About Us page.

8. Use a slider graphic or a motion graphic. Three-window sliders are a nice visual effect that adds movement to the page and delivers on three core procedures or important messages that you want people to know about. Motion graphics are slick and make your practice seem so legitimate.

9. Social media icons are a great tool because it allows potential visitors to see another side of your practice. It's a great place to publish more videos and photos. Also, it's a great place to see how your practice interacts with its community. From an SEO point of view, it helps build your practice's social signal, which is a signal that Google is incorporating into its algorithms.

    Social media is no longer just sexy marketing speak, it is a must when it comes to online marketing.

10. Don't forget about going mobile. Mobile compatibility is huge because mobile search has passed desktop search by a fairly wide margin now in 2019 and will continue that trend through the 2020s.

    The most important rule to remember with mobile is to make it easy and to get all of the important information front and center. Make sure everything is only a click away and always have your click-to-call button on top that gets the patient connected to your front desk.

# CHAPTER 18

## Mobile Optimization

More and more patients are searching for doctors via mobile device. Interestingly, typing searches into Google is still the leading way that people are finding what they are looking for online, but there is another growing trend.

### Hey Siri: Find Me a Doctor!

Research giant Gartner predicts that, by 2019, 20 percent of all user interactions with the smartphone will take place via virtual personal assistants (VPAs).

"The role of interactions will intensify through the growing popularity of VPAs among smartphone users and conversations made with smart machines," said Annette Zimmermann, research director at Gartner.

I've always loved Gartner. They are a powerhouse and I used their research extensively during my time at IBM, Accenture and KKR they are the most respected name in corporate research, which is why you should pay special attention to what comes next:

> *Gartner's annual mobile apps survey conducted in the fourth quarter of 2016 among 3,021 consumers across three countries (U.S., U.K. and China) found that 42 percent of respondents in the U.S. and 32 percent in the U.K. used VPAs on their smartphones in the last three months. More than 37 percent of respondents (average across U.S. and U.K.) used a VPA at least one or more times a day.*

Evidently, Gartner found that Apple's Siri and Google Now are currently the most widely used VPAs on smartphones. Fifty-four percent of U.K. and U.S. respondents used Siri in the last three months. Google Now is used by 41 percent of U.K. respondents and 48 percent of U.S. respondents.

Getting the VPAs to recommend your practice could be MASSIVE for your practice revenue. Earlier this year, we figured out how to implement this for our Elite 300 clients. It's epic.

Gartner further explains:

> *With a predicted installed base of about 7 billion personal devices, 1.3 billion wearables and 5.7 billion other consumer Internet of Things (IoT) endpoints by 2020, the majority of devices will be designed to function with minimal or zero touch.*
>
> *By 2020, Gartner predicts that zero-touch UIs will be available on 2 billion devices and IoT endpoints. "Interactions will move away from touchscreens and will increasingly make use of voice, ambient technology, biometrics, movement and gestures," said Ms. Zimmermann."*

Wow. What does that mean?

It means times-are-a-changing. Mobile smartphones can access websites, as well as perform a multitude of other tasks, which is why they have become more of a necessity than a luxury these days. For you, as a medical professional this provides a unique opportunity to connect with local customers via their mobile devices and have Siri or Google Assistant recommend YOUR PRACTICE!!! The importance of this cannot be overstated.

I won't go into detail here about how this is implemented because we have to save some of our secret sauce for our Elite 300 practices; but, before you start to develop a mobile arsenal to drive more inbound calls via Siri or Google, you must first figure out who your mobile competitors are in the local medical or dental market. It is important to know who you are up against in mobile marketing so you can plan your strategies accordingly.

(If it's one of our Elite 300 practices though, good luck. Ha!)

To effectively do this, you need to identify your closest competitors and learn what mobile techniques they are using to generate their sales.

First, find out which of your competitors have a mobile-optimized website. One quick and easy way to find out is to pull up their website on your mobile phone.

Did it load quickly? Was it easy to find their contact information and other details that consumers tend to look for while on-the-go? If so, they have invested in their business by making sure their mobile customers and prospects are taken care of.

Now, pull up your website on your mobile phone. If it's a nightmare, it's not your phone that is the problem, it's your website. This means you have been losing potential business.

## Text Marketing

Next, figure out which of your competitors are using text message marketing. If your competitor Dr. Petersen is doing it, she is probably telling the world to "Text 123ABC to 212-555-5555." If you see promotions such as this, they are using text messaging to build a list of repeat customers. This is powerful stuff.

In fact, text messages are one of the most cost-effective and results-oriented forms of marketing today. Text message marketing allows practices to draw in local consumers with a great offer. Then, they send out occasional messages or coupon offers to keep them coming back to buy more treatments or procedures.

Let's say one of your patients had plans to contact your practice today after work about an expensive fee-for-service procedure, but they recently joined your closest competitors mobile list and had received a text coupon offer from their practice before they had the chance to call YOUR practice.

Who do you think the patient will call?

The great thing is, you can take THEIR patients as well using this same method and others. There are many other forms of mobile marketing a practice could be using to capture the attention of local patients such as mobile SEO, QR codes and mobile apps.

## Mobile Self Analysis

What is your status when it comes to staying connected with patients consumers using Mobile Marketing strategies? We implement a software that makes it super easy for our doctors to do this, but again, if you can't afford us... listen up:

Researching your competition is a necessary task if your goal is to become the local authority in your specialty practice niche. But, it is equally important for you to analyze where your practice currently stands in order to move forward.

Are you currently running a mobile marketing campaign, but not seeing the results you want? Or, do you want to start a mobile marketing campaign but keep putting it off because you don't know where to begin?

Every practice in your local area is in a crucial fight for more patients and profits. Therefore, in order to enjoy a spike in sales, your practice can no longer ignore the profitability of ramping up your mobile efforts.

Many practice owners in highly competitive, saturated cities like Los Angeles and Miami spend money like crazy in competing with similar practices, while neglecting to take a close look at what they're doing. Analyzing your mobile status will help you figure out which weaknesses are holding you back and which strong points can help you win the war for new patients and big dollars.

You need to understand where your past efforts have taken you, as well as what your future has in store for you based on where you stand today. For starters, it is crucial that you take note of what you are and aren't doing to generate more sales using mobile marketing.

- Is your mobile website user-friendly? Does it load within seconds or take forever to render properly?

- Does your mobile website have all the relevant information on it that consumers look for while on the go?

- Does your mobile website come up high in the rankings on mobile search engines, or is it nowhere to be found when local consumers perform a search for you "doctor + your city" or "dentist + your city" on their mobile devices?

- Have you started to build a text marketing list? If so, what are you currently doing with that list?

- Are you focused on building a trusting relationship or are you spamming them with offers daily and getting high rates of opt-outs?

- Is your opt-in/call-to-action on all your printed and web marketing materials?

- Are you using QR codes as an additional method of increasing awareness about your business?

- Do you have your QR codes on all your other marketing materials? Are you using them to direct traffic to your mobile website?

- Do you currently use a mobile app to keep your audience engaged?

As you can see, there are a lot of things to consider when it comes to making sure your business is on the right track toward beating your local competition with mobile marketing.

## Spy On Competing Practices

Do you want to know how your closest competitors are driving more business by using mobile marketing? Just look at their practice's mobile campaign yourself.

Mobile marketing has recently opened new doors for practices that want to market their products and services by using mobile phones as personal mini-billboards. This has been enhanced by the fact that more and more people own mobile devices, and use them to find local products, services and businesses of all types regularly.

To beat your competitors in the world of mobile marketing, you need to know what they are doing to be ahead of the curve. Digital technology is growing at astonishing rates and is not expected to slow down anytime soon. This alone is causing many companies to be left behind when it comes to new-age technology.

Spying on your competitors' mobile marketing initiatives may seem like a daunting task, but it's not. In fact, all you need to do is identify which are taking-away most of your patients and let the research begin.

You should begin by visiting their mobile websites on your phone. Go through the websites and take note of the look and feel, the features and the traffic flow. Although your goal is NOT to copy exactly what they're doing, you could get a few pointers for your own mobile website.

Next, find out how their text message marketing campaigns operate simply by joining their mobile list. They probably have a text call-to-action placed everywhere, so opt-in and pay close attention to what happens throughout the entire process. This is the perfect way to get a first-hand look at their treatments, procedures and promotions.

Are your competitors using QR codes to generate interest in their practice? If so, whip out your mobile phone and scan their codes to see what lies behind them. Where do the QR codes take you? What type of incentives are they offering to get prospective patients to scan them?

Another thing you can investigate is your competitors' mobile applications. Download their apps and see what they're offering and how user-friendly they are. These are rare in the local-provider health care field, but if you do have a competitor that has one, look out. They have effectively weaponized digital marketing and you could be in for a tough battle.

The information you gain from your research should be used solely to set up your mobile marketing campaign that will not only beat your competitors, but will also attract new patients and keep them loyal to you and your practice.

My former Harvard ethics professor and my good friend who is a professor of ethics at University of Denver would both probably want me to tell you that spying on your competitors is probably not illegal, but there are ethical limits you should observe to remain fair. So, under no circumstances should you use unethical measures to jeopardize your competition in your quest for mobile marketing, nor should you incur any substantial cost on their behalf in your use of their technology.

Also, you should check with your practice attorney to make sure your local laws are followed.

## Get Prospective Patients to Call Your Practice

The secret to beating your local practice competitors is making your practice more interesting to your target audience. There are several ways to do this using mobile marketing if you plan, focus on the right things, and maintain your campaigns over time.

As much as you would like to boot your local competitors out of the picture, the fact is that a few of them might be using some of the same mobile marketing methods as you are.

So, your focus should be geared toward getting your patients choose your practice over theirs. This is easy to do if your efforts are consistent and persistent.

It is up to you which tools you use to work positively toward attracting new customers and keeping the ones you already have. We have some great tools for our Elite 300 clients, but again, your mileage may vary.

Here are a few tips that can work in your favor and help local patient prospects choose you:

- You need to have a good website that is mobile-friendly and easily accessible by mobile phone users in your area. People are using their mobile phones to access the web to search for local products and services while on the go. Make sure your site loads quickly, gives them the exact information they need, and is easy to navigate.

- If you choose to start a text message marketing campaign, make sure your text messages offer great value, relay a clear message, and are short and informative. Also, be sure to send messages out consistently, yet conservatively. Create a careful balance that makes sense for your practice and your target audience. Need a boost in getting new mobile subscribers? Give your practice and prospects a great incentive for a treatment or procedure in exchange for opting-in and watch your list grow exponentially.

- Consumers love businesses who stay "on top" of the digital age. They expect you to have a website, to actively involved in their favorite social media outlets, and to be easily accessible from their mobile devices. Implement the use of QR codes to keep your local consumers engaged and provide them with "instant gratification."

- Mobile SEO should be used effectively to attract qualified traffic to your website. Mobile users search for local products and services constantly on their mobile devices when on-the-go. If your practice does not rank in the results, there is major potential-patient-profit-leak left for your competitors to scoop up.

Now that you have your website conversion fundamentals in order and have a proactive Mobile Marketing plan, you can start to think about Social Media Marketing.

## CHAPTER 19

## Social Media Marketing

There is a lot of BUZZ around Social Media (Facebook, Twitter, Instagram, Snapchat, YouTube, LinkedIn), but how can it be leveraged by a medical or dental practice?

In this chapter we are going to cover social media marketing for your practice. I hope that by now, you've learned a lot about how to position your company online, how to rank well on the organic listings on the Google Map, and how to rank well in the organic non-paid-listings. Now, we're going to talk about social media marketing, and how you can utilize social media tools like Facebook, Twitter, Instagram, Snapchat and LinkedIn to grow your business.

As I talk to doctors throughout the country about Internet marketing and social media, I tend to get a puzzled look. The question is, "How in the world does all of this social media stuff apply to my business? How can I possibly use Facebook in a way that would help me grow my revenues, grow my service calls, and get more repeat business?"

I'd like to try and bridge the gap on where the "low hanging fruit" is for social media is in your medical or dental practice by asking, "What's your number one source of patients today?"

Just stop and think, *where does most of your revenue come from?*

**You'll quickly conclude that your number one source of practice revenue is repeated and referral business.**

Mr. Nicholas Shawn Chavez

The lifeblood of any service business (including health care) is existing customers (patients) returning for services (procedures) over time, and those existing patients referring you to their friends and family. If social media is harnessed correctly, it gives you the ability to take that repeat and referral business and take it to a whole new level.

Let me explain why I feel that it's a great place for you to really connect with your customers and get more repeat and referral business. Just a couple of Facebook stats:

> The Facebook currently has 2.41 billion users as of Q2'2019 and at one time, the average user had 135 friends, and checks in between 6 and 9 times per day, studies show that those numbers are increasing annually.

If you can get your real customers, current and past, your sphere of influence, to connect with you on social media, Facebook, Twitter and/or Instagram your business is exposed to their 135 friends as soon as they "like" and follow your page.

It's almost as if they'd sent an email, or they'd sent a text message out to all their friends saying: "I saw this great doctor in our area. The next time you need a similar procedure, why don't you think about them?" It's extremely powerful for your practice to gain exposure to their sphere of influence and it's dead-simple to execute.

Another major advantage is that they've given you permission to remain top-of-mind with them. As I said, the average user checks in between 6 and 9 times per day. They login to check out the updates on their Facebook wall and to see the updates of all the companies and people they have liked or are friends with. If you're posting updates to your social media profiles, the people who have liked your page are going to see the new content whenever they login.

They are going to see an update and your practice logo. They're going to see some special offer or promotion, and it's going to peak their interest. Next time they need a procedure or a treatment, who do you think they're going to call? You, that's who!

After they see you once, there is an even higher probability for them to use you again, and refer you to their friends, because they remember you and had a good experience with your staff. They know who you are. You've remained top-of-mind.

If you look at major companies like Coca Cola, Pepsi, and Frito-Lay (all former clients of mine), they spend billions of dollars a year on advertising and promotions: TV, radio, web & print. Why?

They're developing their brand, so they can maintain what we call "TOMA," top of mind awareness. Leveraging social media inside your existing sphere of influence is a great way to tap into that top-of-mind awareness.

Where should you start? Where can you start using social media, with all the different platforms out there? With so many different social media tools, what should you be using?

Earlier, we talked about having a blog and putting out consistent updates. Well, blogging ties very nicely to your social media strategy. These are the social media profiles you want to have set up and ready to roll in your practice.

Let's talk strategy before we get into the granular details. Talk about high level. How do you leverage social media and how do you gain that initial following?

First, you'll want to utilize email to get initial engagement. Having an active social media profile with daily updates isn't worth much if you don't have likes or viewers, right?

Now, at the same time, if you have thousands of irrelevant people that have pressed like on your website or on your Facebook profile, it's not going to work to your advantage if they're not people in your area. They're not wealthy enough to afford your procedures or treatments and they're not the target market that we discussed in the marketing fundamentals.

You want to make sure that you have a strategy to get your real patients and your true service area engaged with you in social media. You should leverage email to engage your patients to get to your social media profiles. We recommend a multi-step process:

The first thing you want to do is build that list or go into your customer relationship management system, (let us know if you need one, we have one that works amazing for practices and it is SUPER reasonably priced), and export the name and email addresses of your patients. Current patients, past patients, sphere of influence of your friends, your business partners, the people that you do business with, and put them into an email.

Queue up a nice little message that says, "Hey, we appreciate your business. We appreciate your relationship over the years. We're getting active in social media and would love to have you engage with us. Please go to Facebook.com," and give them a direct link to your Facebook page, "and press the like button."

There are a couple of things you can do. You can offer them an incentive, something of value like a coupon or a discount. Or, if you feel like you've got an active patient base that knows who you are and likes you, just ask them to do it as a favor.

You'll be able to start building that following. Now, you don't want to stop there. You don't want to just send one email out that says, "We're on social media." You now want to build it as part of your business.

In the Google Maps Optimization section, I talked about having an email go out after service, thanking the customer for their business and asking them to go ahead and write a review for you on one of the various online directory sites. (Our CRM automates this, it's pretty slick.)

Well, there's no reason you couldn't send a subsequent email to that contact, maybe a day or two days later, that says, "By the way, we're actively involved in social media and would love it if you would engage with us." Then give them a direct link to your social media profiles where they can press like, subscribe, and follow to start engaging with you on social media.

The key is that it needs to be an automated process where you're typing your patients' names and their email addresses. These emails go out to everybody that you serve without any hiccups, without any potential for dropping the ball. If you don't do it consistently, you won't get a true following and you won't get your real patients engaging with you on these social media platforms.

That's step one. Leverage email to build that initial engagement and that following of your real customers. Remember, we want authentic customers, and not just throwaway links and subscribers.

Once you've got that part squared away, you have got to think about what you are going to post:

- What information are you going to put up and how frequently?
- You should post to your social media profiles once a day.
- If that seems like too much for your practice, post once a week at a very minimum.

These should be informative posts. It should not be a sales

pitch. It should not be, "Here's 10-percent off your next service."

You can make an offer every third or fifth post and then but more than 60-80% of the time it should just be social content: "Here's a picture of a smile that we reconstructed", "This is what's going on in our city", "Here's a picture of us at the latest trade show.", etc.

Keep it informational, keep it relevant, keep it social, and then you must engage. Social media isn't a one-way dialogue. You shouldn't be going to your social media profiles and pushing out updates that don't have any engagement. You shouldn't just be posting. You should be trying to get people to reply to your post: "Hey, that was funny", or "That's a beautiful picture", or "Thanks for that great tip," all of which you can reply to.

Then, listen to what your fans are saying. Once you've got a flow – you've got 50, 70, 100 or a couple of thousand people that have liked you – you are going to be able to hear what they are saying as well. They might post something that's totally irrelevant to you, like "Hey, tomorrow is Barbara's birthday!" There is no reason that your organization couldn't reach out and say, "Hey, wish Barbara a happy birthday from us!", from your company. They will think, "Wow, this is a practice that cares. This is a company that's real and authentic."

Engaging in social media is probably the lost art. Most people that use social media just post one-way messages, which is not the idea. It's a social platform, so there should be conversation. There should be dialogue.

The next thing you want to do is to develop your brand and make sure that you enhance the bio section on each one of these profiles. Within Facebook, Twitter, LinkedIn and Instagram you will have the option to fill in an 'About Us' or bio section. Write some interesting information about your practice there.

Take the information from the 'About Us' page on your website where you talk about where your practice was founded, why you started the practice, the treatments and procedures that you offer, and pop that into the bio section on your social media profiles. Easy peasy.

You also could put an icon on each one of these social profiles, and you want to make sure that you're using an image that represents your practice. It can either be a head shot of the lead doctor or it can be your logo.

If your personality represents your brand, then it's not a bad idea to use a nice head shot so that people resonate with you. People tend to buy from individuals more than they buy from businesses because a business is an anonymous entity and a person is someone that they feel they can get to know, like and trust.

It's all about branding, so make sure that you're leveraging the header graphic and the image icon. If there is an option for you to customize the background, do it! You want to make sure that you've got the elements that marry up with the overall branding of your practice.

Make sure everything on your social media profiles is consistent with your website. On your website, you've got a color scheme, a logo, and maybe you've got brochures that are made up. Make sure that there's a consistent flow, look, feel, and color scheme on all your social media profiles, website and offline materials.

Don't forget to have a plan:

- How often are we going to post?
- What types of posts are we going to put out there?
- How are we going to engage our patients?

- What social media profiles are we going to be involved with?

Remember earlier when we talked about the fundamentals of your marketing plan (market, message & media)? You need to make sure that you have a clear understanding of who your current patient is and who your ideal patient is. Then, make sure that you are crafting a message that will resonate with that ideal patient. You need to think about all these things as part of your social media strategy, because consistent effort here is the ONLY way to change the composition of your practice and the associated revenue.

If you are super excited to get to work, please don't just dive in.

A common mistake would be to just setup the profile and start posting with no thought process or plan behind it.

Think about it:

- What pages are you going to be on?
- What message are you going to put out?
- What color scheme are you going to use?

Set all of that up and then get very specific about who your target is. Is your ideal patient the wealthy type? Is your ideal client a golfer?

One solid method is to schedule your post types:

- **Monday, Wednesday and Friday** are the days that you are going to put up tips associated with your treatments and procedures such as: what to do when a patient gets a surprise acne outbreak or what to do in the event of an emergency sunburn or why a patient should consider Botox.

- **Tuesday and Thursday**, you'll post photos of interesting things relative to your practice: pictures of before-and-after reconstructed smiles, or pictures of a client that lost 60 pounds during treatment, or a patient who is smiling at his wedding after a successful rhinoplasty.

- **Saturday and Sunday** you can post special offers.

I am not advocating this specific editorial calendar you should follow. My point is to make it easy on yourself or your staff to know what is going up and when. It can be streamlined and it can be automated.

When we talked about the blog in the SEO section, we went over leveraging content. Because that content is king, you must be creating updated information on a consistent basis. This content can go up in various places. As you post a new piece of content, it can go to your Facebook and Twitter pages automatically. It can go straight out to Pinterest if it has a photo included, and you can take your blog content and syndicate it to recreate great social media content.

Remember, content isn't necessarily just written text. You are an expert on your craft. You can either sit down and write about it, you can take an audio recorder and record yourself talking about it, or if you're comfortable on video, you can break out the camera phone and shoot a video talking about an issue that your ideal consumer may be facing.

That one piece of content can serve multiple functions. The first function can be posting videos up on the social media, on websites like YouTube, Snapchat, and Instagram, where you can upload interesting clips and videos.

Again, you can also take that video and have it transcribed using a service like otter.ai. There are various transcription services, but that one is pretty good and it's free for the first 600 minutes per month. Now that video of you talking about the benefits of drinking enough water for clear skin and weight loss can now be transcribed into text, which may then be used as a blog post and be syndicated into your social media profiles for your patients to read. Another step beyond that is using that same audio and turning it into an audio podcast that you can have hosted on your website.

There are a lot of things you could do to take your content and work with the modality that you're most comfortable with. Some doctors like to write. Some doctors like to talk. Some doctors like to be on video. Figure out what you are most comfortable with and run with that. This is how you create social media content for your online marketing plan.

Remember, educational content that's published in multiple places gives you industry expert status. By publishing and getting picked up in the AMA/ADA, the local newspaper or a reputable blog, you are considered a published expert. This is going to further drive your credibility, which in turn, will result in more referrals.

**What not to post:**

1. Use the 80/20 rule for marketing messages, put out 80% information and 20% marketing.
2. Keep it business related. Your political and religious beliefs are never a good mix with business.
3. Photos of your kids playing tee ball are good, but don't let it dominate your practice page.
4. Keep your vacation photos on your personal social sites.
5. Keep your non-practice related opinions, beliefs, and interests to yourself.

Sometimes knowing what not to post is more important than knowing what to post, because the natural tendency is to go to these social media profiles, and just post promotional material. So, don't post a treatment-coupon every single time you log in. If you do that, everybody that liked or subscribed to your page will start to disappear before you know it. They'll stop subscribing, they'll unlike you, and they'll unfriend you.

## When and How to Engage

We talked about asking your patients to "like" you on Facebook, and asking your patients to write testimonials. We also talked about interaction and responding to your patients' actions. "Hey, thanks so much for the follow. We appreciate it." Or, if they write you a testimonial, make sure you promote it.

Not only should you thank them for their testimonial, but you should also share your appreciation.

"Hey, Mike, thanks so much for the positive testimonial. We appreciate your feedback. We appreciate your business, and this is what keeps us going. We love to help and heal people." Then, you could take that testimonial and put it on your website or embed it on your website through the various widgets and short codes that Facebook provides.

If you do this regularly and correctly, you're going to grow a nice following of real patients in your true service area. You're going to remain top-of-mind and it's going to help you grow your practice in terms of the lifeblood of your organization, which is repeat and referral business.

## Notes From the Facebook Front Line

Facebook is quite possibly the single most efficient, accessible, and lucrative tool in existence right now. With well over 2 billion users, it's a cost-effective way for healthcare practitioners to become local celebrities if they know how to use the tool properly.

DigitalGoals' job is to provide you with the know how to use Facebook to help grow your practice revenue by 300% in a HIPAA compliant way. It's a tall order. There's no way we could consolidate the Facebook expertise needed to triple practice revenue into a digestible chapter of a book.

If you've seen the movie Moneyball, the story of how the Oakland A's used statistical analysis to ascertain which low-budget players would make them a viable contender in the MLB, you'd have realized that statistical analysis or experience and intuition alone doesn't win games. You must have both.

The digital world and your newest crop of patients grew up together, and our social team lead has worked in SEO and digital marketing since he was old enough to legally hold a job. This puts DigitalGoals me in a unique position to help you.

Our technologists are at once the 70-year-old grizzled baseball scouts, and the young ambitious number crunchers trying to get you the best "moneyball-esque" deal on your Facebook Ads.

First the basics, then the secrets. Let's start by making you aware of the Facebook family, which consists of:

- Facebook
- Instagram
- Messenger
- Audience Network
- WhatsApp

In order to advertise with the Facebook family you need to create a personal profile. Once you have a personal profile, you can create a page, and once that page is created we recommend building it out to the greatest extent possible. This is going to be how you are represented to potential and existing clientele, so look sharp!

You might feel the urge early on, when that '0 Likes' or '0 followers' number is staring you square in the face, to start inviting people that you know to come and like or follow your page. If they are not existing clientele, please refrain, as this will later skew your data.

You must be very careful; Facebook is a complex series of algorithms and you need to be a granular level technician if you want to triple your practice revenue with it. Facebook is only as good as your data, so protect it the best you can.

We do would, however, encourage you to join or create groups that are relevant to your business. What we are doing here is creating as many digital avenues as possible for people to find you.

Once you feel as though you're in a good place with your page, you'll want to navigate over to Facebook Ads Manager. This is where you will live out of. This is where the game is played.

Here you will set up campaigns, which contain ad sets, which in turn contain ads. At the campaign level you'll choose from the following ad objectives:

| Name | Objective | Associated Reporting Metric |
|---|---|---|
| Brand Awareness | Displays your ad to people that are most likely to be interested in your service | Estimated Ad Recall Lift |
| Reach | Shows your ad to the maximum number of people | Reach |
| Traffic | Drives people to your website, your mobile app, or Messenger | Link Clicks |
| Engagement | Increase post engagement, page likes, or event response | Post Engagement |
| App Installs | App Installs | App Installs |
| Video Views | Shows content to people who are most likely to watch it | 3 Second Video Views |
| Lead Generation | Allows people to share their contact info with you | Leads (Form) |
| Messages | Encourages people to have a conversation with you in Messenger | New Messaging Conversations |
| Conversions | Asks people to do something in a website or mobile app | Conversion Event |
| Catalog Sales | Link to images of every item you sell, and Facebook will display different ads to different people based on how they've engaged with ads in the past | Website Conversions |
| Store Traffic | Encourages 'brick and mortar' visits | Store Traffic |

Then, at the Ad Set level, you'll be asked to select your:

| Name | Types | Variables Contained |
|---|---|---|
| Target Audience | Core Audience<br>Custom Audience<br>Lookalike Audience | Location<br>Age<br>Gender<br>Languages<br>Demographics<br>Interests<br>Behaviors<br>Connections and Advanced Combinations |
| Placements | Automatic Placements<br>Edit Placements | Facebook:<br>News Feed<br>Marketplace<br>Video Feeds<br>Right Column<br>Stories<br>In-Stream Video<br>Instant Articles (FIA's)<br><br>Instagram:<br>Feed<br>Explore<br>Stories<br><br>Messenger:<br>Inbox<br>Stories<br>Sponsored Message<br><br>Audience Network:<br>Native, Banner, Interstitial<br>Rewarded Videos<br>In-Stream Videos<br><br>Functionality:<br>Specific Mobile Devices<br>Specific Operating Systems<br>Exclude Content<br>Exclude Publishers<br>Exclude Gaming Live Streams |
| Delivery Optimization | N/A | Optimization for Ad Delivery<br>Cost Control<br>When You Get Charged<br>Ad Scheduling<br>Delivery Type (Standard/Accelerated) |
| Budget | Daily<br>Lifetime | N/A |
| Schedule | N/A | N/A |

Finally, at the Ad Level you'll choose your:

| Name | Types | Variables Contained |
|---|---|---|
| Identity | N/A | N/A |
| Format | Existing Post<br>Carousel<br>Single Image/Video<br>Collection<br>Instant Experience | N/A |
| Ad Creative | N/A | Image/Video/Slideshow<br>Headline<br>Description<br>Website URL<br>Build a URL Parameter<br>Ad Card Automation<br>Primary Text<br>Display Links |
| Tracking | Conversion Tracking<br>Facebook Pixel<br>App Events<br>Offline Events<br>Optional URL Parameters | N/A |

The correct combination of these variables may well put you on a path to growing your practice revenue. You know your clientele better than anyone, which makes for a good starting place.

However, if you allocate all of your ad spend based on intuition alone, you might be sorely disappointed with the results; which is your first goal should be high-value audience data aggregation.

This is the business goal tied to our first campaign.

Using this, we can figure out the objective that will yield the most useful results. Remember, we want to find out as much as possible about your audience, and when it comes to statistical analysis, there is strength in numbers. The greater the number of people we source information from the more accurate our results will be.

Your gut might tell you to go for a Reach campaign since it will serve the highest number of impressions, but that won't provide high-value trackable data. So instead, a Traffic campaign that directs to your website will likely be your best bet. We'll call this first campaign "Target Audience Split Test".

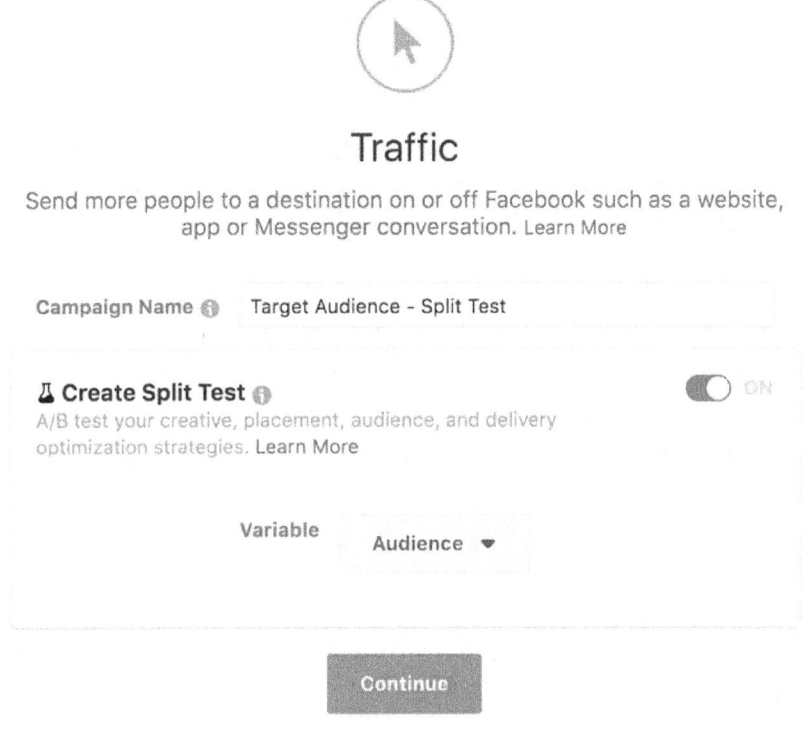

Split tests are a low budget way to determine correlations (not causation) between identity and buying interest. You'll be able to use split tests to identify the variables that perform better to meet the macro-objective of increasing practice revenue.

The variables you can test are:
- Audience
- Creative
- Delivery Optimization
- Placement

For the purposes of this example, we will only be talking about split testing for target audience. However, all of these, excluding placements, should be tested in your first three weeks; roughly one week per variable. Placement doesn't need to be tested because the Facebook algorithms for automatic placement are better than any manual process we could conduct.

Split testing will create multiple ad sets. Each ad set should be identical in every way except for, in this instance, the audience that you are targeting. This means that the creative and delivery and placement should be constants across your ad sets.

You'll want to be sure that the Facebook Pixel is integrated with your website and you've set up an offline conversion API that can communicate with your results page. This will help us measure who is interested in your service. If you've already had these set up for a while then you'll have a leg up on data aggregation and can likely start doing more nuanced split testing from the jump.

You know your practice better than anyone, so I would recommend creating five to ten different ad sets each containing an archetypal identity of your high value patients.

**It bears mentioning that you should not, under any circumstances, upload your patient information directly to a custom Facebook audience and create a "Lookalike Audience" from it.**

It blows my mind that has to be said at all, but there are "spikey haired Internet marketers" out there that recommend this very practice. This action is not HIPAA compliant and, in a time, when cybersecurity tactics are changing by the hour, doctors simply cannot afford the possibility of a Facebook-wide data hack exposing patient data and their unwise exploitation of said data.

So, using data other-than your actual patient list, run these ads simultaneously for 4 days using the same budget for each ad set and an impression frequency cap of 2 impressions every 4 days. Facebook will recommend a budget that you should use in order to achieve accurate results. All other delivery optimization variables should remain in their default settings for this campaign.

Now it's time for the ad itself.

Remind yourself that your business goal is *high value data aggregation*. We want the kind of creative that will give us the most insight into your potential clientele. The creative that does this the best is custom video. You might remember this from when my dad had touched on authority ramp marketing and SEO.

The reason why custom video will give us high-value data is because we can measure the percent of the video that was viewed by each target audience. As you can see, this is an example of a highly detailed funnel that provides multiple pieces of data which we can then use to assess the proper variable settings for your practice.

After you've run this test for four days, Facebook will send you an email telling you which ad set performed the best along with a confidence level that comes in the form of a percentage. The minimum confidence level that we would consider to be reliable is around 75%.

Now, your competition might be doing this, but because they aren't thinking about all the data in this critical manner, so most of them will make a misstep here. They will see the audience that performed the best and then they will focus their attention on that audience. This is a poor use of your time and money.

A smart marketer would use the Ads Reporting tool in Facebook Ads Manager to view the audience overlap of successful results in each ad set and then compare it to the custom audience that will be created via click throughs (tracked via the pixel) and the percentage of their video watched.

Next, you'll want to split test creative and delivery optimization.

Congratulations! You've taken the first step in defining your target audience and it will continue to get more refined and more accurate the more campaigns you run.

This is an example of something you could do for new general patients, but imagine if you picked the three most profitable procedures that you perform and underwent the same process, so as to deliver a very personalized message that yields high ROI for you.

Now we're talking.

Let's discuss now why it benefits you from an economic standpoint to invest in high-value audience data aggregation.

Facebook ads are shown to Facebook users using an auction.

Facebook is constantly preforming a balancing act in their effort to maximize advertiser value as well as optimize their consumer experience. This is good news for you, because it means *that the winner of the auction is not necessarily the ad with the highest monetary bid, but the ad that creates the most total value.*

In other words, the more relevant Facebook predicts an ad to be to a person, the less it should cost the advertiser to show the ad to that person. We won't bother with the technical explanations of the algorithms used to calculate total value or all the technicalities of how Facebook determines the winning ad, but if you're interested, our interpretation of the most rudimentary version of the equation can be found below:

[Advertiser Bid] * [Estimated Action Rates] + [User Value] = Total Value

If you're doing this on your own it may behoove you to investigate the technicalities of the auction at some point, but for the purposes of this book we'll simply give you the 12 guidelines we use for staying competitive in the Facebook auction, and getting optimization events for less money:

1. Bid based on your willingness to pay for conversions after calculating your break-even point of the specific ROI you need for profitability

2. Enable targeting expansion

3. If you're optimizing conversions, optimize towards the highest intent event that has the most data

4. Enable automatic placements

5. Turn on campaign budget optimization

6. Pay attention to the user experience. Monitor your feedback and improve your landing page. After your ad is served more than 500 times it receives a daily relevance score from 1-10. The higher the relevance score, the better it's considered to be performing.

7. Being specific with targeting

8. Refreshing your ad if it's saturating the audience

9. Learn from testing to see what works

10. Avoid using offensive or misleading content

11. Improve the quality of your audience by constantly asking yourself if you are excluding in the most strategic way possible for the data that you have available

12. Use the 'estimated daily results' tool to make more informed delivery control decisions

This is a fairly-primitive version of the Elite 300 Facebook patient acquisition plan, but it's the only one that you would be able to realistically implement while continuing to run your practice in place of simply hiring trained professionals to implement it properly.

A trained professional would set up the campaign, execute, evaluate and then continue to execute and evaluate until they've achieved the most efficient results given the budget. That being said, the nuance and detail and improvisation skills a trained individuals such as those folks on the DigitalGoals team would have acquired in order to accomplish the tasks properly are the result of very hard work and long hours.

Facebook is an incredibly complex tool that appears to be a simple one, making it dangerous for anyone who is foolish enough to underestimate it.

This short section about Facebook Ads barely scratches the surface and there are a multitude of approaches and tools and techniques not discussed here; however, if you've recently graduated medical or dental school and have gotten your practice license, this should be enough to get a few patients through your doors so you can start paying your loans back in earnest!

## CHAPTER 20

## Video Marketing

The key to the Elite 300 program is getting recurring patients through video marketing through our "Patients for LIFE" efforts.

Did you know that YouTube is the 2nd most used search engine (ahead of Bing & Yahoo)? Most doctors and their marketing directors are focused on search engine optimization but neglect the opportunities that video and YouTube provide.

Implementing a Video Marketing Strategy for your practice can get you additional placement in the search results for your practice keywords, enhance the effectiveness of your SEO efforts and improve patient conversion.

There are several reasons that you should engage in video marketing for your contracting business. The primary reason is that it's going to increase your exposure on the search engines, giving you more placeholders for the keywords that are most important to you. It's going to enhance your SEO effort by driving great visitors to your website and creating relevant links to your website, improving conversion. Once somebody gets to your website, if there is good video on the home page and the subpages, that is going to resonate deeper with your potential patients. It will help convert those visitors from just browsing around page to picking up the phone and calling your office.

There are significantly less videos than there are web pages on the Internet. So, creating relevant and quality video content for YouTube and other video sharing sites is a huge opportunity.

These videos will help you to connect with patients and answer their questions when they're looking for information on what you do.

I talked about the fact that you can now show up in search engines with an image next to it, and you can obtain multiple place holders on Google for the keywords that are most important to you.

If you do this right and you optimize your videos correctly (I'm going to showing you exactly how in this chapter), you can start to have your video show up in the natural search on Google, which is extremely powerful. It also gives you the opportunity to have more placeholders, for the various procedures that you provide.

## Video Helps with Your Overall SEO Effort

The other thing that we can accomplish with video is the enhancement of our SEO efforts. As covered in the SEO section, links are critical for ranking. By creating good video content, you could drive inbound links to your website from high level video sites like YouTube, Vimeo, and Metacafe.

Again, you don't want to have just the generic Home, About Us, Our Practice, Contact Us pages on your website. You want to have a page for each of your core treatments and procedures. Videos that link to those pages is going to help with that SEO effort. Also, you're going to find that video content on your website, and on the pages of your site, reduces your bounce rate and improves the metric of visitors' time on site.

These are SEO factors. "Bounce Rate" refers to somebody getting to your practice page and clicking back immediately or browsing away. Google understands those actions as the page not being relevant to that search. Not good.

If the majority of the prospective patients that get to your site click off and leave right away, your bounce rate is high, and Google is going to start to show you less prominently in their results. That's part of the Google algorithm. The other factor is the amount of time spent on the site. If somebody gets to your practice site, stays there for ten seconds, and then moves on, the visit might not get treated like a bounce, but Google is looking at the length on the site.

If you have a video and a visitor takes the time to watch it in its entirety, that's improving your website visit length statistics. Even if they only watch a couple seconds of the video, you have captured their attention long enough that Google is going to see that your site is relevant. Very good.

Don't get confused by the notion that having video on your page automatically improves your SEO. That's not necessarily the case. But, having people stay on your page longer and not bounce off does impact SEO positively. It's going to give you better search engine optimization because you get the links from the video sites, you're improving your time on site, and reducing your bounce rate. The other benefit of video that is probably even more powerful than anything, is that it's going to improve prospect-to-patient conversion rates.

You can have the best SEO strategy in the world by driving hundreds of patient prospects that are looking for your treatments on a daily basis; but, if it's not converting and if prospective patients aren't picking up the phone and calling to book a consultation for your treatments and procedures after they visit your site, you're missing a major opportunity.

Having intelligent video on your site is going to improve conversion.

Video clips resonate with people. They like video because it gives them the chance to get to know and trust you before they call you, especially if you follow my personal strategy rather than creating a very clinical type of video. If you create authentic video of your team, the practice owner or your associate doctors talking directly to the camera, connecting with patients on an emotional level, answering questions and giving a strong call to action... your patient conversion rate will improve.

It also gives you the ability to connect with different modalities. Everybody thinks in a different way. Some patients are readers and will read all the content on a page. Some patients are listeners, so if there's the opportunity to listen to something rather than read, they'll choose to listen.

Other patients like something visual. By having video on your website, combined with text (I'm not saying to abandon text), you could connect with every type of person. Some people will watch the video and only connect with that, because they wouldn't take the time to read a plain text web page.

We understand that video is powerful, it's going to improve your SEO, it's going to help us get better placement on the search engines, and it could potentially help with conversion. How can we expand upon this?

What we want to do is create simple videos about your practice, your procedures and the most frequently asked questions. You are then going to upload those videos to YouTube and other video-sharing sites, and syndicate them to your website and social media profiles.

What type of video should you create? Like I keep saying, "People resonate with people." Keep it simple, be real and be personable. Put your real face on the camera, or the face of someone that represents your practice. Be frank and to the point, it doesn't have to be a 20-minute video, an appropriate length would be 30 seconds to 3 minutes long- just enough to get the message across.

## What to do with your video content

What are you going to do with the videos once you've got them? Now that you have completed shooting your videos, what you want to do is setup a YouTube channel.

You can do this by going to YouTube.com. You want to upload your video, name it correctly and intelligently, putting it in terms that will be likely used to search this type of content. If a patient is looking for a root canal, they are going to type in "your city root canal." You want to name the video using your keywords. When you upload it to YouTube, you want to title it "Omaha root canals" or "Omaha endodontic therapy" and then put a description with a link to your site. "Visit us online at yourpractice.com/rootcanal" and then include a description about what you do, briefly outlining what was said in your video.

## Some YouTube Best Practices

When you setup your channel, make sure that you give it a "city plus procedure and name of your practice" title, instead of just your company name. You are also going to add tags with keywords to it. Don't just leave the tag area blank.

Make sure you use your name, address and phone number in every description on your YouTube channel because this is a good citation source.

As covered in the Google Maps optimization chapter, citation development is critical (having your company name, address and phone number referenced consistently across the web).

Mr. Nicholas Shawn Chavez

This is a great place to get citations. Also, make sure that there's an image avatar with your practice logo. You can update the default image by putting in your logo or put a picture of the team or office.

Here's some visual representation of this. If you log into YouTube and create your channel, you'll get an email confirmation. Once you're set up, you can go to the "My Channel" settings and make some of the updates I referenced on the previous slide.

To change your logo, simply click "change" and choose your image – a very simple step.

Where it says "Your company name," it's going to default to something basic such as your email address on Google. You can hit "change" and update it to say "your city Endodontics" or "your city Dental" and then a dash and your practice name.

This gives you the chance to get your YouTube channel itself to show up for your keywords in the search engine. You will also could add your channel keywords. That is where you can type in words such as "your city dentist," "your city orthodontist," "your city braces," and of course your practice name.

From there, there's a section where you can click "About" and put a description about who you are, which procedures you do, and what geographic areas you serve. You can get as creative with this area as you want, but it is most important to make sure you first put a description of your services, and your city.

If you're in Nashville, you put Nashville. If you're in Houston, you put Houston. If you're in Phoenix, you put Phoenix. Put your phone number and, again, restate your name, address and phone number. Citations are important. Having this in the description area is powerful citation source.

Always put your name, address and phone number the same way as you did on your Google Map listing, your Angie's List listing, etc. That way, you will be consistent across the web, improving the probability of ranking in the Google Map listings.

Now, let's talk about video tagging best practices. Let's say you created the inventory of videos I recommended: an intro video and clips for each of your services.

How did you tag those videos to maximize the opportunity and to make sure that you're going to rank well in search?

- Title Video with City Service – Practice Name (always mix this up a little)

- Description should always start with http://url.com and then describe the service using those same keywords. ALWAYS ADD N.A.P. INFO AT THE BOTTOM OF THE DESCRIPTION

- Use your keywords as tags and include the practice name

- Choose most appropriate screenshot

- Click "advanced settings" and add address to video

The first thing you want to do is have your primary keywords in the title of the video as well as a description that includes the "http://" before your web address.

In the description area, you can put in "We're a full service XYZ type of practice. We serve this area. This is our name, address and phone number," but at the very top, you should have your practice website address, including the "http://".

If you just put www.yourpractice.com, YouTube won't understand the link and it will show that it isn't clickable. If you put "http://" the link will be clickable, and visitors will go straight to your page, and they also get the link authority from having that link back to your practice website.

Choose the screenshot and add video. Whenever you upload your video you can control your title and your description, as well as the ability to add tags.

Again, don't call your videos "your practice name." Don't call it "root canal." Don't call it "endodontics." Call it "Your city + that service," and then your practice name. Title your videos the same way that somebody would search.

If it's your intro video, you might want to call it "your city + your primary procedure/treatment" Ex. you're a local "Cleveland Dentist for Root Canals."

It is critical that you have the right titles on your video. It is what is going to make it so that Google can locate it and include it in search results.

The next thing you want to do in your description is to put the link at the very top. The first thing you want to do is include a link back to the home page or to the specific page that you're discussing in the video.

If it's the teeth whitening page, don't put a link to your home page. Put a link to that teeth whitening page, and again "http://yourpractice.com" -- make sure you've got that "http://".

Below, you add your tags. Within those tags you can put in your city dentist, your city orthodontics, your city endodontics and everything in between.

**What else can you do with your videos?**

Now that you've updated your video and you've properly optimized it, your title is correct, and your description is posted, how else can we use these videos? Where are we going to leverage them? Well, to really get the benefits of that conversion component, we need those videos to be posted on our website and social profiles as well.

The best way to do this is to copy the "embed code" and post the videos right on your site. The intro video should be embedded on the home page and the service-specific videos should be posted on the appropriate subpages. The way we do this is right within our YouTube channel or YouTube account.

Go to the Video Manager and find the list of all the videos that you have. Choose the video that you want to post on your website and choose the share and embed option.

You will then be provided with this little piece of code, and that's what I have highlighted on the screen. It goes from I frame to I frame. This is the specific code for that video. If you are updating your website on your own, copy and paste the code right into your website's HTML. If you have a detached web manager, send the code off to them with details on where you want it posted.

Once the code is embedded in your HTML, it will show up on the page itself. That's what we really want to do with these videos. And, of course we don't have to limit ourselves to YouTube. There are a lot of very well-known video sharing sites out there.

Mailchimp is a service I have personally used and recommend. It's easy to use and offers similar features to Constant Contact. The interface is clean and easy to use.

## What to Send and How Often

First, what do I send? You must use the 80/20 rule, 80 percent good information and 20 percent sales. If all you send is emails about what procedures you offer, your patients will never read it. It's a great way to kill your email list and alienate your patients.

Draft up some information about your medical or dental specialty, give good healthy living tips, throw in some self-care / home-care tips, and make sure it's information that will help your users. For the 20% of your emails that are in-effect sales pitches, add a coupon or a special price you will honor. If you don't want to discount, consider offering a gift card to your patients for referring their friends and family.

The cadence of your email-sends is very important. I recommend 1-2 emails per month and sent around the same time every month. It is important to commit to a date. More than twice a month is too much and annoys patients. I get an email from a company I purchased from in the past and get 3-4 emails a week from them, 100% sales, sometimes several times a day. I removed myself from that list *with a quickness*.

## Get & Stay Legal with Video Email

Ensure that you build in a mechanism that allows your patients the option to "opt-out" of receiving email messages at the bottom of every message. Make sure that it's easy because nothing is more annoying for your patients than receiving emails that they don't want. It can also devalue your brand as a trusted, busy doctor.

If someone does not want to receive your messages, then remove them from your list. Don't obsess over it or take it personally, as they may be getting emails from too many sources and just want to clean out their email box. Rest assured that it does not mean they will stop visiting your practice.

Again, you want to leverage HIPAA compliant email marketing as part of your overall Internet marketing strategy. The best way to use it is to be sure you're collecting opt-in email address from all your patients and prospects. From there, use email marketing to get online reviews for your practice, engagement on your social media accounts and remain top-of-mind as a strategy to get more repeat and referral patients.

## CHAPTER 21

## GoogleAds Profitability

In this chapter, we're going to talk about Pay-Per-Click Marketing on google to help you understand how it works, why it should be integrated into your overall practice expansion strategy, and how you can run a really effective program that can drive consistent, profitable patient flow for your practice.

**Why PPC should be part of your overall online marketing strategy**

- It's the quickest method for patient acquisition. You can start a program within a few days. (Patients NOW.)

- Show up as often as possible where your patients are looking while you get your organic SEO in place.

- Show up for non geo-modified terms, such as "doctor", "implants", "Botox injections," etc.

First, PPC gets revenue quickly, unlike a long-term SEO program, setting up your website, building links and having the right on-page optimization. The SEO process takes a little bit of time to materialize. What you do today and tomorrow, will start to pay dividends via organic Google search results in three to four months.

With PPC advertising, you set up your campaign and will start to see your practice ads serve in just a few days. It can drive great revenue, especially during the times when you need to make sure you're taking in enough revenue to grow your practice.

You want to show up as often as possible when someone's looking for your services. Having a pay-per-click ad that appears on top of the organic search results, on the map-money box, and to the side of the organic results section is important. With PPC, your practice can show up multiple places and significantly improve the chances of getting your ad clicked on. Essentially, a PPC campaign gives you that additional placeholder on the search engines on page one.

Ads also give you the opportunity to show up for keywords that you're not currently ranking for in your organic SEO efforts. These are what I like to call non-geo-modified keywords. With PPC, your practice can appear in search results for non-geo-modified keywords (e.g. doctor, orthodontist, plastic surgeon, ophthalmologist, oncologist, cardiologist). You can constrain the search results to be shown only to people within a 10-to-25 mile radius of your office. If you're in Miami and somebody searches within that area for "dentist" or "general surgery," you can set the parameters so that Google only shows your ad to the prospective patients that are searching within that geographic area through what Google calls "geofencing" which is how Google identifies IP addresses and further isolates where the search originated.

Google can also determine who ran that search, where they ran that search from, and then place the ads based on the advertisers that are set up for that area. You only pay on a per-click basis, but you're able to show up for those keywords in those major markets.

Another reason that you want to consider running a pay-per-click campaign is because you can run mobile PPC campaigns. With mobile PPC campaigns, when a prospective patient is searching for specialty procedures from a mobile device, it's typically because they need immediate service; this means that they're not as apt to browse multiple pages or listings. Now, if a prospective patient runs a search on their mobile device, and you have a pay-per-click campaign set up, that search will be PPC enabled. Patients can simply hit your ad and rather than browsing to your website and researching, the ad can automatically dial your front office number to book an appointment.

On a mobile PPC campaign, you're paying per call as opposed to paying per lead. It's very powerful, and these are the reasons you want to have PPC as part of your overall Internet marketing plan.

## The Google Ads Auction Process

Let's review how Google Ads works. In the simplest sense, you're paying on a per-click basis and you can choose your (e.g. doctor, orthodontist, plastic surgeon, ophthalmologist, oncologist, cardiologist). As you pick those words, you bid and you pay on a per-click basis.

So, let's just say you're bidding on the keywords "San Antonio Dentist," and there are a lot of other dental practices in that city that want to rank for that keyword. If you say that you'll pay $2.00/click and your competitor says that they'll pay $5.00/click, they're going to be at the top. Assuming nobody else has placed a higher bid, $2.00 is going to be ranked second and $1.20 is going to follow. The fact is that you pay on per-click basis and you are bidding against your practice competitors to determine how your practice will rank for your keyword(s).

The ad buys function as an auction, just like if you were to buy a nice Patek Phillipe watch on eBay. People are bidding and whomever can offer the most money is going to win the auction for the top position.

With that foundational understanding, we can now explain why most PPC campaigns fail. What tends to happen is a lot of pay-per-click campaigns are built on the notion that the highest bid wins. So, doctors pick their keywords, enter the highest bid-per-click and hope that everything turns out the way they want it.

**Why Most Pay-Per-Click Campaigns Fail**

- Practices setup only ONE ad group for all services (e.g. teeth whitening, dental implants, full arch replacement, root canals, etc.)

- Practices don't use specific text ads and landing pages for groups of keywords

- No strong call to action or OFFER on the landing page

Typically, practices setup only one ad group for all services. Your practice should have one ad group instead of different ad groups for each type of service. Also, there aren't specific text ads or landing pages for those ad groups and groups of keywords.

What you wind up with is the same landing page and the same text ad, whether your customer typed in "dentures," "emergency dentistry," "teeth whitening," or "six-month smiles" in the search engine. Whatever was typed into the search engine was likely very specific and should match up to a very specific landing page, but that doesn't generally happen for the practices that are attempting PPC campaigns on their own. All the ads usually just direct to the practice's home page. With this strategy, not only is your practice PPC campaign going to convert poorly, but your cost-per-click will also to be higher.

The other reason why most pay-per-click campaigns fail is because there isn't a strong call-to-action on the landing page. So, you were just charged $5.00 or $9.00 to get a potential patient to your website and the page isn't even compelling because it does not have a strong call-to-action.

It doesn't tell the potential patient what to do next. If you factor these common reasons why pay-per-click campaigns tend to fail, you can better prepare yourself and set your practice up for success in the way that you execute your pay-per-click marketing.

## Understanding the AdWords Auction Process

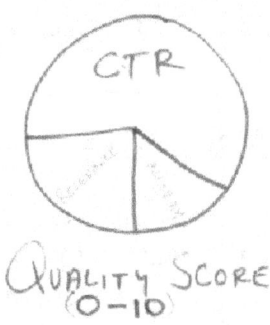

$$\text{ACTUAL CPC} = \frac{\text{AD RANK TO BEAT}}{\text{QUALITY SCORE}} + \$0.01$$

| Advertiser | Max. Bid | x | Quality Score | = | (Ad Rank) | Actual CPC |
|---|---|---|---|---|---|---|
| Mary | $2 | x | 10 | = | 20 (no. 1) | 16/10 + $0.01 = **$1.61** |
| Tom | $4 | x | 4 | = | 16 (no. 2) | |

Let's talk about how the Google Ads auction process actually works because it's not as simple as the highest-bidder winning. It's more complicated than that. The reality is, Google needs to feature the most relevant results because their endgame is to get people to keep using their search engine over the competition. This is their definition of quality control and customer retention.

Google has historically been great at maintaining their 80%

share of the Internet search market through a relentless focus upon relevancy. The second they sacrifice relevancy for dollars, is the second they start to lose their pole position in the search market.

So, Google had to figure out a way to make their pay-per-click program grow around relevancy. And so that's why they established the ad-quality score. They needed to make sure that the ad that had the most relevancy gets a higher quality score and as result, can have a lower cost-per-click.

The way I like to explain it is, if I go to Google and I type in "BMW," obviously I am looking for a Ferrari dealer or for information about a new Ferrari. Lamborghini could say, "That's our demographic also. If someone types in Ferrari, they're looking for an exotic sports car and they are likely in the market to buy. Why don't I bid on the keyword Ferrari?"

There is nothing to stop them from doing this; however, the person that searched for Ferrari isn't necessarily looking for a Lamborghini. So Lamborghini could say, "I'll pay $25.00 for everybody that clicks on me when they search 'Ferrari'."

But, Ferrari might say, "That's my brand and I am going to compete for it, but I am not going to spend $25.00 for every click on my own brand. I'll pay a dollar for every click." Based on the ad quality score, Google may decide to serve Ferrari because it's in the best interest of the person researching the brand, the consumer. It's also in the best interest of overall relevancy. That's how quality score works. Quality score is really driven by three core components

- **Click Through Rate**

- **Relevance**

- **Quality of Landing Page**

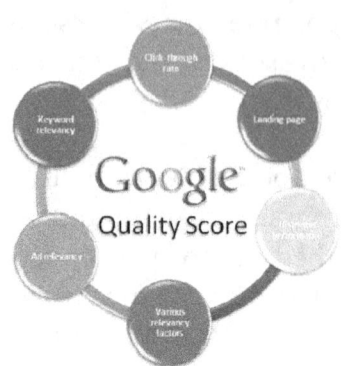

- Click Through Rate
- Relevance
- Quality of landing page.

As somebody conducts a search and your website shows up on the page in the pay-per-click section, Google is tracking what percentage of those people saw your ad and clicked through. That's one of the primary metrics that they analyze. So, if your ad is relevant, if it speaks to the person's needs, and if it's compelling enough to them that they click through, Google just made more money per-click. This will make them willing to give you a higher quality score because you've got better click-through rate.

Also, relevancy is a major factor. How relevant is your text ad to the keyword that was typed?

For example, if a prospective patient types in "carpal tunnel Denver" and your text ad reads

"We're a rheumatology practice in the Denver area,"

vs.

"We specialize in carpal tunnel syndrome here in the Denver area. Click here for to book an appointment to help with the pain."

Which do you think is more relevant to the prospective patient? Google wants their search results to be as applicable as possible. They're looking at your ad click-thru rate, they are looking at the relevancy of your text ad to your keywords, and they are looking at the quality of your landing page.

If your landing page (the page that you drive people to) doesn't match up with what the person just clicked based on your text ad, or if that landing page doesn't have a strong call-to-action and the person quickly returns to the search engine, that signals to Google that your ad was not very relevant, which will result in a quality score reduction.

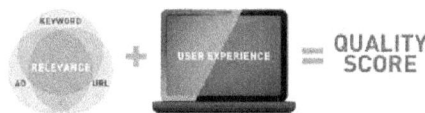

## Better Quality Score = Lower Cost Per Click for Top Positions

By having a higher quality score you can bid lower and still achieve the top position. This is where you can actually win in the pay-per-click marketing game because a better-quality score results in a lower cost-per-click for those who hold the top positions.

Again, if we just look at the reason most pay-per-click campaigns fail, it's because:

- Your practice only set up one ad group

- Your practice had the opportunity to create a separate ad group for each one of your core treatments, but you don't use a specific text ad that's going to compel a potential patient to click and improve your click-through rate

- Your practice doesn't have a strong call-to-action that matches up with what the potential patient was looking for

- Your practice doesn't have a high click-through rate, relevancy, or an applicable landing page.

All these issues result in a lower quality score and, by extension, you're going to wind up paying more per-click. PPC marketing is very competitive. If you're paying more per-click, then you're not going to be able to spend that much because you won't be getting enough calls to generate return on investment - it's some very unforgiving math.

## How to setup your PPC Campaign for Success

Let's talk about how to position your pay-per-click campaign for success. What can you do to ensure the highest probability of success in your pay-per-click campaign? For starters, set up ad groups based on the specific groups of services that you offer.

Write compelling text ads that are relevant to your specific treatments and procedures. Then, link your ads to the specific pages on your site rather than the home page, making sure that the specific pages on your site that talk about that service should have a strong call.

The other thing you want to pay attention to is exact match versus broad match. You have a setting inside your Google Ads campaign where you specify whether you want Exact Match or Broad Match. Always elect to do exact match. The reason is because if you choose broad match, you could very easily find your practice accidentally showing up on the search engines for a lot of keywords that have nothing to do with your specific practice.

The other thing you want to do is pay attention to negative keywords – keywords that you don't want show up for in the search engine. A great example of this is, jobs, employment, marketing, etc. If someone types in "your city dentist," that's great. If they type in "your city dental jobs," that's somebody looking for employment in dentistry. Unless you are trying to fill a position or if you want to use your pay-per-click budget to get applicants, it's probably not the kind of the person you want to attract.

Setting up negative keywords means, for example, if someone types in "jobs," "employment," or "marketing services" anywhere in their search, it pulls your practice's Google Ad out of that search so you won't be paying for clicks from somebody that's not relevant to your bottom line.

## Mobile PPC Optimization

I talked a little bit about making sure that you've set up mobile pay-per-click campaigns. I've mentioned the major transition of people searching on their mobile device versus people searching on their desktop or laptop computer.

More and more people are accessing the Internet via smart devices; their iPhone, Android, and tablets. The searcher is typically in a different mind-frame when they are searching from a phone rather than from the computer. When you're searching from a phone, you often just want to get the information right away, and/or want your problem solved as soon as possible. You can set up a campaign to have click-to-call built into your mobile campaign. In the image above there was a search conducted from a mobile device, "Dallas Dentist".

The patient will see a "Call" button towards the bottom? That's what we call a mobile PPC campaign with the click-to-call function turned on. If somebody hits that "Call" button, they're connected immediately to that dental practice location. This is a quick alternative to having to search for the website and the phone number on their own. Plus, you can see on a mobile phone there is not a lot of screen space. Those pay-per-click listings become prominent and they dominate the search results page on mobile. A lot of times, you're going to get the majority of the clicks if you're in those top two positions. It's all about convenience, and the click-to-call function allows that.

It's extremely powerful to connect with these people that are searching from mobile devices. Set up a mobile-specific campaign and choose "Mobile Devices Only." Then you can pick your geolocation. That would be your 10-mile or 25-mile radius. You then click a button to turn on the *click-to-call* function. That's how you wind up with a pay-per-click campaign that has you in the top positions if bid on correctly, with the options for prospective patients to do a *click-to-call*.

Just to recap, you want to set up your ad groups correctly. Make sure that you pick keywords that group them together, you write text ads that speak directly to that group of practice-relevant keywords and ensure your landing page (where you are sending those specific searches) speaks to the text ads and the group of keywords. You also want to be sure that you have some type of strong call-to-action that prompts your prospective patient into calling your practice as opposed to pressing the "Back" button and looking at four or five other practice competitors in your city.

As the relevancy of your ad groups campaign and your keywords improve, your cost-per-click will decline and your conversion will improve. You can spend less and still get better positioning and more traffic to your website. This is how you maximize the profitability of your pay-per-click marketing campaigns and succeed in PPC where others fail.

# CHAPTER 22

## Pay-Per-Lead Programs

Let me say right up front that this is very, very dangerous territory and I do not recommend the practice to any doctor who is serious about HIPAA compliance. Is it legal? It seems to be if everything is done properly and your business associate agreements (BAAs) are airtight and you trust your business partners.

If you decide to do this, please remember that I've sternly warned you against doing so.

With that warning in mind, let's review the procedure:

With pay-per-lead services, medical and dental practices can contract with an outside organization who is placing ads on Google, Facebook or Instagram with the goal of luring prospective patients to divulge private information (some of which is undoubtedly protected by HIPAA) to be resold to medical or dental practices who will contact the prospective patient and convert their need into a procedure and the associated revenue.

Some short-sighted health professionals like this very much because they can pay-for-performance, which is to say that the prospective patient must fill out all the information that the practice needs to "close" the sale for the procedure without having to "waste the time" consulting with the patient. This is of course, folly.

Here are three great reasons that you'd probably want to steer clear of a service like this (if you can even find someone crazy enough to want to do this for your practice):

1. The leads are very expensive. Think $200-500 per.

2. While you may have signed an exclusive agreement for the lead, there is no way for you to ensure that your lead broker has not sold the lead to a competing practice.

3. There is no real way to determine the chain of custody for the medical information that you are receiving, if there is a HIPAA violation, the practice that performed the procedure is going to have their door knocked first.

Some of these lead brokers are offshore, so they don't fear the US Department of Health and Human Services or our Department of Justice and they can (and do) collect fresh leads for medical and dental practices. Think this through, do you really want a partner who does not have to answer to the same organizations that could hold your feet to the fire? That this is "risky" behavior is putting it very mildly. Still, I've met a great many dentists and physicians who are all about the dollars and the biggest houses and boats that they can buy.

We won't work with those doctors. Sure, we like money and it's our primary goal to increase revenue; but, we will only do so in a legal, ethical and sustainable manner.

Some non-U.S. doctors may be reading this book, and if they do not have a law similar to HIPAA in their country, then if may be a valid manner of acquiring great patient leads.

International doctors can pay either per lead or can pay on a per-monthly basis to gain access to all the leads that fall within your geographical market or service area. Again, check your local laws and know that this process is a risky one; but, if you need some additional leads or you've got an killer inside sales team that can follow up and close the patients while getting a credit card and scheduling the procedure purchasing leads may be a profitable option for your practice.

I'll stop short of recommending any of these services directly to international doctors because we do not work internationally, our Elite 300 practices are intended to be 100% U.S. based.

If this method of patient acquisition is of interest to you, there are an abundance of these types of services. The best way to find additional lead services specific to your practice would be to run a Google Search.

## PPC vs Pay-Per-Lead (PPL) services

This is important to talk about regardless of whether a practice is paying per lead or just conducting a PPC campaign. The magic is in the follow-up.

I guess if I were to search for a benefit in the risky pay-per-lead service world, it would be that you only pay your marketing company when they send you a qualified lead.

If you have followed the plan outlined in this book, you should have your organic keywords ranking well in the search engines and map listings, proactive social media, email marketing and a well-structured pay-per-click marketing campaign. If you want to bump the lead flow, these pay-per-lead services can help to start channeling new people that are in the market for your procedures.

Note that you MUST be diligent and quick with your follow up if you choose this route. There are countless horror stories about how badly these lead services work. If you have built your Internet marketing strategy on pay-per-lead services, you're destined to fail. You can't build a sustainable business around just this one strategy; but, if it's an add-on to a an already strong Internet marketing program, then it might be relatively effective. Just know that these leads are likely to be composed primarily of price-conscious shoppers. They are using these services because they want to get the lowest price possible. Keep that in mind.

If you don't have the time and energy or the front desk / inside sales staff to chase leads, then I would say to pass on pay-per-lead services altogether. Reason being that these leads may also go out to a number of other practices in your area, so you have to be aggressive. Your team usually must be the first person to get customers on the phone and you have to be professional with a compelling offer that makes them want to choose your practice as opposed to the competition.

You also need to setup a follow-up system to make sure that you have a fallback plan in place for leads that you can't reach right away. You can get these leads in a variety of formats. They'll send you an email, you can log in and download an Excel list, or you can receive a text message that alerts you as soon as the email comes through.

If you have an appointment scheduler on your team, be sure to assign this person specifically to follow up on leads so long as he or she is a decent salesperson. Know who is accountable for these leads when they come in. If it's going to you, to your scheduler, or even one of your front desk team, you don't want there to be any confusion about who is responsible for following up because then the expensive lead slips away and you lost money.

Specifically assign someone the responsibility of reaching out to these people. Have a predefined script on how the call should be handled. Be professional. Be courteous. Be quick.

Whether it be PPC or PPL, many of these procedures are going to go to the first practice that gets the prospective patient on the phone, so it is important to be somewhat aggressive. Don't just call once; have a process in place where you reach out to these people 3 to 5 times over the course of the subsequent 24 hours because they're in the mindset to buy.

You should have a contingency plan in the event that you don't get the prospective patient on the phone. If you don't get them on the line, make sure that you're taking note of their name and their email address so that you can remain top-of-mind with them.

A practice in your service area that is competent in this specialty procedure is going to book the revenue, so it might as well be YOUR practice.

If you're not sending an email follow-up, and if you're not adding them to your email marketing database, then you're wasting marketing dollars. If you've just spent $50, $100, $250 for the PPC or PPL, and you're not proactively and diligently following up with them via email, you might as well take your ball and go home.

Below is a script of a solid fallback strategy. Set up an email auto-responder on a program such as MailChimp or Keap, where your scheduler can enter the patient's name and email address, and have a series of emails that go out to the customer over the next several days. Remember not to let this be your crutch. Don't think that these emails are going to do the trick.

We recommend a CRM to our clients that does much of this for them and is HIPAA compliant. Reach out and let us know if we can help you with it.

Anyway, back to the email:

 Email 1 – Subject – Your Recent XYZ Procedure Inquiry

Patient Name, you recently submitted a request on [PPL / PPC Site] regarding your interest in an XYZ Procedure. I called and left a message for you on the number that was listed and look forward to talking with you soon. You can reach me directly at xxx-xxx-xxxx. With so many XYZ practices to choose from in the [YOUR CITY], I know it can be hard to know who you can trust. At ABC Practice we have been serving the [your city] area since 1982 and are dedicated to resolving your XYZ issue quickly, cost effectively and without leaving a mess. Give me a call at xxx-xxx-xxxx to schedule your appointment.

Email 2 – Special Offer for XYZ Procedure

Patient Name, you indicated that you were in some need of some XYZ Procedure a few days ago. I'm sure you have received a number of calls from us at ABC Practice because we are eager to earn your trust. WELL – as our outside-of-the-box approach to getting your attention, we want to offer you a special offer. If you call us today and reference this coupon, we will grant you 10% off your procedure cost.

<ATTACH COUPON IMAGE>

Call now and get 10% off your XYZ procedure with ABC Practice.

Email 3 – Subject – RE: Your Recent Procedure Inquiry

Patient Name, I hope this note reaches you well. You reached out to us earlier this week via [PPC / PPL site] looking for some help with your XYZ Procedure. We would love to be of service to you. I have tried you a few times on the phone number you listed with no success and don't know if you are just busy or if you already booked an appointment with a different doctor here in [CITY]. Please shoot me a quick reply to let me know if we can be of assistance, or give me a call at xxx-xxx-xxxx. Thanks, Dr. Brody

It's the aggressive follow up work on the phone that is going to get you the business, not the email sequence. But, these templates are great to have in your lab coat pocket as a fallback strategy.

Again, don't stop in the first few days. Now you've got their name and email address presumably on an opt-in basis. You should be marketing to these people via email at least monthly. You should have an email database of patients and prospects that you should be sending out emails to once or twice a month with some type of update.

"Here's what's going on with our practice. Here's why you should consider this procedure NOW because of this special offer incentive." This is to remain top-of-mind so that you can build your patient-base both in email and social media.

As you look at PPC and PPL services, be cautious. Don't overspend.

Put phone number tracking in place to make sure your practice is getting a strong return on its investment.

# CHAPTER 23

# Track, Measure AND Quantify

Now that you've built and optimized your practice website, you've got an ongoing link building strategy in place where you're creating inbound links and moving up in the search engines, you have implemented email marketing and social media marketing initiatives, and have possibly implemented a paid online marketing campaign including PPC, you need to put some tools in place so that you can track, measure and quantify your data to ensure that you're marketing dollars are generating activity.

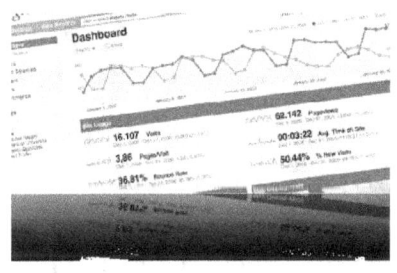

- Google Analytics
  www.google.com/analytics
- Keyword Tracking Report
  www.gshiftlabs.com
- Call Tracking Report -
  www.callfire.com

There are a great many different tracking mechanisms that you can put in place. I'm going to recommend three core tracking mechanisms, the first being Google Analytics. Google Analytics is a fantastic website data analysis tool and it's completely free.

Google Analytics will show you specifically:

- How many visitors visited your website on a daily, weekly, monthly, and annual basis
- What key words they typed in to get there
- What pages on your website they visited

- How long they stayed

The primary data point you'll want to examine from Google Analytics is how many visitors interacted with your practice website AFTER you started your SEO / PPC campaign? Remember that SEO takes a while to yield, so don't be disappointed if the numbers are a bit low in the beginning. Take this data as a benchmark and use it to compare to future data on an ongoing basis.

Ultimately, what you are looking for is whether or not the number of visitors to your website is increasing and whether or not they are becoming patients. Is your primary metric (revenue) moving in a positive direction?

To examine this, you can also set up reports within Google Analytics. You will need to verify that you own the website through an electronic process initiated by Google, and then you install a small piece of code into your website's HTML. After you have done that, you've got the Google Analytics tracking in place and you can begin benchmarking.

## Keyword Tracking

The second mechanism that I recommend is keyword tracking. Near the beginning of Part IV, we talked about keyword research to determine which keywords prospective patients are typing in when they need your services. If you followed along, you came up with a list and all those keywords were combined with your cities and sub-cities to make geo-referenceable long tail keywords lists.

There are tools that will tell you how you're ranking on Google, Yahoo, and Bing for those various keywords. A few options include:

- Bright Local
- Raven Tools
- SEMrush

The keyword tracking tool I recommend is called BrightLocal. You can learn more about it at www.brightlocal.com. There is a somewhat substantial cost associated with this service, but it is great resource for tracking your search engine optimization progress. To use it, you'll take your keywords, put them into the BrightLocal Keyword Tracker and then set up a weekly and monthly report that shows where you rank on Google, Yahoo and Bing for your most important keywords.

With a report like this, you can easily see how your website is trending in the search engines.

If you've built out the website correctly with the right on-page factors (title tags, H1 tags, meta descriptions, etc.), if you're building links, developing citations and have a proactive review acquisition system in place, you'll see yourself move up in the results. When you see yourself stagnating, you can go back to that keyword, figure out which page is optimized for it, look at your links and link profile, and whatever is necessary to push that keyword to the next level.

## Call Tracking

We talked a little about this in Chapter 10. Having better rankings and more visits to your website is great, but these are really vanity metrics if they aren't associated directly with patient acquisition; and a practice cannot generally acquire a patient until a phone call is made. Calls are what drive practice revenue. You want to have some type of tracking mechanism in place to know how many calls are coming in from prospective patients on a monthly basis and what's happening within those conversations.

Then you must figure out if the calls are turning into sales? That's where the rubber meets the road. That's why we're doing all of this. Who cares if you're in the number one position if it doesn't result in dollars to the business?

There are a number of call tracking tools that you can use; but make sure the one you choose is HIPAA compliant.

Most of these call tracking services will let you choose a phone number based on your area code. So, you type in the number you want to get. Then, you can take that tracking phone number and you can put it on the graphics on your website so that you can track the number of calls and even listen to recordings of the conversation.

You can report on the number of calls using the Internet and play back recordings of those conversations. It's extremely powerful to know the number of calls you were getting when you started versus the number after you incorporated your new marketing strategy, or else how will you measure growth?

You can go in and listen to these phone conversations with your front desk and ascertain how many of those calls turned into booked appointments while knowing what the revenue associated with that service is. That is how you get a true gauge on the ROI associated with your online marketing strategy.

## CHAPTER 24

## Next Steps

Hey, nice work. You finished the book!

Hopefully, if you are running an already successful practice, you just skipped over Part IV in its entirety to figure out how we can work with one another. Doing this work yourself promises a massive learning curve, sleepless nights and wasted funds.

Just a quick recap on what we covered and where:

- **PART I: Plan**

  - In Part I we discussed the mindset of the doctors with whom we choose to work, we talked a little bit about my background and why some very successful doctors have chosen to trust our team at DigitalGoals.

- **PART II: Build**

  - In Part II we discussed the right way and the wrong way to engage vendors to help in the build out of your practice. We talked about what a coach is and methods for evaluating their trustworthiness, we also touched on other Internet marketing companies out there in the medical and dental space and how they may be violating HIPAA on behalf of their medical and dental clients. I finished Part II up with some contextual information about PPC, Social and SEO so you could understand a bit more about how we serve our Elite 300 practices.

- **PART III: Acquisitions**

  ◦ In Part III we discuss using the additional funds generated from Internet-marketing-based-patient-acquisition to fund the purchase of additional practice locations to grow your annual top line revenue into the 7 or 8 figure range. We also talk a little bit about what you'll need to think about if you are looking to sell your practice and the other professionals (accountants, lawyers and bankers) who can help you make your dream a reality in a risk-adjusted manner.

- **PART IV: Everything you never wanted to know about Internet Marketing**

  ◦ I sincerely hope you didn't read this section in detail, but I am hopeful that you at least skimmed it. In Part IV we discuss at a medium-level of detail the steps one must take to implement an Internet marketing program for one's practice. I suspect that this section will be read hungrily by two groups of people: students who are still in medical and dental school and competitors to DigitalGoals.

  If you are the former, we wish you the very best of luck in starting your practice. Give us a call when your income stabilizes and we can help you own your service area for your specialty when you are ready to do so.

  If you are the latter, good luck. DigitalGoals is dominating the landscape. The only way to beat us is cheat us and it hasn't happened yet.

Either way, if you have taken action and followed our instructions, you should be well on your way to a better knowledge base than you had prior to opening this book.

## Need More Help?

If you've gotten to this point and feel like you need some extra help to implement these ideas, we are here to support you. As experts in helping to grow medical and dental practices across, we have had tremendous success implementing these strategies. You can call us directly with any questions that you might have. Our team will review your entire online marketing effort (Website, Competition, Search Engine Placement, Social Media, etc.) as well as your competitive landscape in your geographical area and come back to you with a complete assessment of how you can improve and what you can do to take your practice to the next level and hopefully increase your revenue by 300%.

## EPILOGUE

Your metamorphosis has begun!

Whether or not you realize it, you have already completed the first evolutionary step to making your practice a success that could produce dynastic wealth.

By reading this book you've re-established yourself as a lifelong learner. Doctors who are lifelong learners naturally find more success-granting-information than doctors who are content to hang their fancy degrees on their walls while wallowing in idle self-satisfaction.

Your decision to read to this book was important confirmation that you are a person of action, who has a desire to have a real impact on your family's life by providing them opportunities that only excess monetary resources can bestow.

I'm calling that fact out and laying it plain for you to realize how important it was that you took action to better yourself and take a brave step on behalf of your family who already admires you because you have the capability and wherewithal that they do not. They believe in you, admire you and trust you to do the right thing to advance their collective life with you.

That seems like a lot of pressure, and the journey can be lonely; but you are <u>not alone</u> for the simple reason that when you finished reading this book, you joined a group of doctors who did the same.

It is my best hope that you join them in the satisfaction that comes from a well-planned career as a doctor with a multitude of patients and the extreme wealth that tends to accompany it.

We have a hidden Facebook group that you should join to chat with other doctors and dentists about the successes and failures that come along with building dynastic wealth through the expansion of a medical and dental practice.

I am quite happy to surround myself with the brilliant men and women here in the United States who have earned the right to call themselves "doctor." It is my privilege to coach and guide them to greater success as they coach and guide me to greater health.

These efforts will take the balance of my natural life to complete properly, and as I'd previously mentioned: being a coach, mentor and friend is my very favorite way to spend time.

I hope I can spend some time being yours.

Respectfully,
Nicholas

Mr. Nicholas Shawn Chavez

## AUTHOR'S NOTE

I launched my speaking career at the age of 5.

At least, that's the story my mother tells me. Evidently, she dressed me in little grey suit, a starched white shirt and a crimson tie for my big day where I was to give a talk in front of my school. She doesn't remember the topic and neither do I; but she said I did well and she was proud. I guess I felt comfortable, so I did it again. And again. And again.

In middle-school I started winning competitions for extracurricular speech events. I'd take the prize money and update our old Packard Bell 486sx with the latest components; I loved the virtuous cycle of learning that speaking created in my life.

My speaking later gave me the confidence to audition and perform in a few local commercials with banks and amusement parks. I won the prize for Second-Runner Up for Talent of the Year for the International Modeling and Talent Association (IMTA) in New York in 1994. My younger brother took first place in New York, and my friend Jessica Biel won IMTA Talent of the Year in Los Angeles in winter of the same year. Our agent had a big year in 1994 and went on to "break" a few other great talents.

Then, I grew up.

Kids, houses, cars, payroll, vacations, lawyers, obligations. Reality was absolutely sucking me dry as it does to a great many of us around middle age.

Then, I met a new friend.

We had dinner with he and his wife at their lovely home overlooking an impossibly green golf course with the majestic Rocky Mountains as a backdrop. They taught us how to play Shanghai Rummy; it was a total blast.

I almost won!

After we played, he invited me into his library and offered me a copy of the book he had recently authored. He then told me how he is paid $10,000 per engagement to speak at colleges all over the United States; he had distilled the content of his book into a one-hour keynote speech that resonated with college students.

I had to do it. I wanted the adrenaline and engagement that speaking in front of a crowd offered; so, I wrote this book and I'm so glad I did.

Money aside, every time I give a speech, I end up meeting fascinating people. A good number of the people I meet very much deserve stage time of their own due to their own remarkable accomplishments in the field of medicine or business. I make it a point to stay in contact with these individuals after the event because they teach me as much, if not more than I have taught them.

For this reason, I often waive my speaking fee entirely.

A speaking fee is nice and insofar as it is available in the event budget, I will most certainly accept it with great humility and appreciation; but, I wouldn't turn down the opportunity to speak to and open a dialogue with other educated individuals like doctors and dentists.

To do so would be the height of short-term, arrogant thinking.

I have talks prepared for:

- Cybersecurity in Medicine
- Protecting Yourself from 3$^{rd}$ Party HIPAA Violations
- Three Steps to a Multi-Million Dollar Practice
- Rich Docs: How to WIN financially by working with Medicare, Medicaid and Insurance companies

So, if you are holding an event for a group of doctors, dentists or students who are going into a specialty in either of those professions; I encourage you to look me up regardless of your event budget. While I do expect that the engagement might yield a client or two for DigitalGoals, I do not intend to "sell from the stage."

The worst part about paying $3,000+ to attend an industry conference is the expectation that you will be educated, but instead you are being pitched the whole time.

I've been to those types of conferences. Believe me.

I have a passion for teaching and connecting with people. I suspect when I finally retire, I'll end up either in politics or academia, trying to educate and make life generally better for the many.

Until then, give me a call. I'd love to help you out with your medical or dental conference speaker line up.

## ABOUT THE AUTHOR

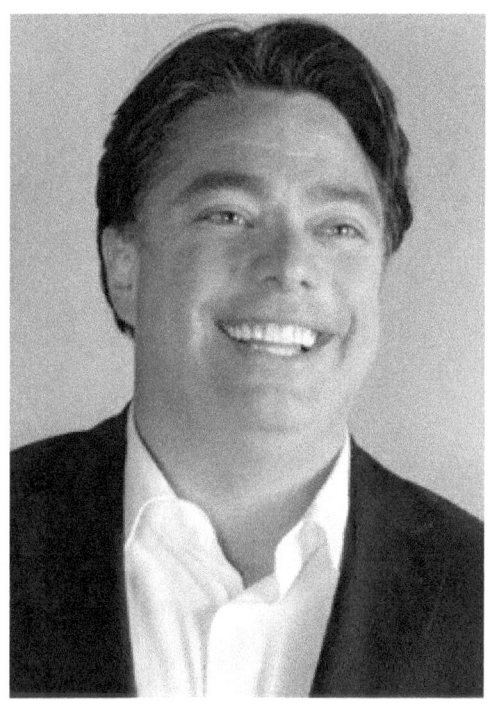

Nicholas Chavez is the host of *The Billionaire Whisperer* podcast; additionally, he is the Managing Director of DigitalGoals, the CTO of bitcoinR and the Founder of Plutocratic.

With a technology career spanning over 20 years, Nicholas has built, maintained or implemented applications and electronic marketplaces as a contractor for the U.S. Department of Defense as well as for some of the world's largest corporations such as Accenture, IBM, Dell, Nestle, JP Morgan Chase, PayPal, AIG and KKR.

He began working for IBM as part of his high school's Gifted & Talented program prior to becoming a technology entrepreneur and achieved a net worth of over $40 million before his 28th birthday.

As of May 2020, Nicholas shall be twice degreed from Ivy League institutions having then earned his undergraduate and graduate degrees from Harvard University and Brown University respectively.

Mr. Nicholas Shawn Chavez

You can learn more about Nicholas Chavez and his wonderful team at www.digitalgoals.com.

# Notes

[←1]
I've never really removed an appendix. That's the point.

[←2]
These results are hypothetical and may not reflect your practice's success. We absolutely cannot guarantee that you will achieve this, or any level of financial success via our services.

[←3]
The price had been reduced to a still-lofty $8 million prior to being removed from the market prior to this book's publication date.

[←4]
This townhouse, despite its insanely high price is a fairly simple 4,500 +/- square foot home in a fantastic neighborhood. It's construct is certainly not Vanderbilt-esque, but the price tag is reflective of the parabolic rise in Manhattan real estate values over 30 years, even if they've been somewhat depressed as of late due to aggressive tax policies at the municipal, state and federal level.

[←5]
Jes & I have never really identified with "rich kids" nor do we want our children to identify as or with such. I'm not advocating creating multiple generations of "trustafarians," I'm simply pointing out that a doctor following the system could likely create dynastic wealth if he or she put the effort in.

[←6]
I do not partake of the water because of all of the plastic in the ocean, but again I digress.

[←7]
These deals seemed so seductive at the time but looking back they were utterly cringeworthy and it pains me that I was arro-

gant and foolish enough to waste time, energy and money on them.

## [←8]
This wasn't as difficult for me as some of the other kids since my nose is of considerable size and gave me a bit of distance from the linoleum floor and I could pick up some decent speed.

## [←9]
Multipliers are all over the place, and can be as high as the mid-teens for specialty practices like LASIK, etc.

## [←10]
These five principles are just a taste of the wisdom the book contains. Buy both Schmidt's book and the Dalio book I mentioned. They are both phenomenal reads.

## [←11]
I am not disparaging inherited wealth. Many of the listeners of my podcast *The Billionaire Whisperer* are members of "old money" families. The preparatory actions of the patriarchs and matriarchs on behalf of their children are to be lauded and praised: for an idle human is often an evil one.

## [←12]
McDonalds wasn't even founded until 1955.

## [←13]
We didn't end up doing a deal because I would have had to become a licensed real-estate professional in order to profit share and I simply do not have the time.

## [←14]
Yes, this guy DID actually write that advice in his book. I own a copy.

www.ingramcontent.com/pod-product-compliance
Lightning Source LLC
Chambersburg PA
CBHW060824220526
45466CB00003B/964